Treating the Critically Ill Patient

The *Essential Clinical Skills for Nurses* series focuses on key clinical skills for nurses and other health professionals. These concise, accessible books assume no prior knowledge and focus on core clinical skills, clearly presenting common clinical procedures and their rationale, together with the essential background theory. Their user-friendly format makes them an indispensable guide to clinical practice for all nurses, especially to student nurses and newly qualified staff.

Other titles in the *Essential Clinical Skills for Nurses* series:

Treating the Critically Ill Patient

Philip Jevon
RGN, BSc (Hon), PGCE, ENB 124
Resuscitation Officer/Clinical Skills Lead
Honorary Clinical Lecturer
Manor Hospital
Walsall
UK

Consulting Editor
Dr Jagtar Singh Pooni
BSc (Hons) MRCP (UK) FRCA
Consultant in Anaesthesia
and Intensive Care Medicine
New Cross Hospital
Wolverhampton
UK

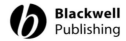

© 2007 by Philip Jevon
Except Chapter 9 © 2007 by Blackwell Publishing Ltd

Blackwell Publishing editorial offices:
Blackwell Publishing Ltd, 9600 Garsington Road, Oxford OX4 2DQ, UK
Tel: +44 (0)1865 776868
Blackwell Publishing Inc., 350 Main Street, Malden, MA 02148-5020, USA
Tel: +1 781 388 8250
Blackwell Publishing Asia Pty Ltd, 550 Swanston Street, Carlton, Victoria
3053, Australia
Tel: +61 (0)3 8359 1011

The right of the Author to be identified as the Author of this Work has been
asserted in accordance with the Copyright, Designs and Patents Act 1988.

First published 2007 by Blackwell Publishing Ltd

ISBN: 978-1-4051-4172-7

Library of Congress Cataloging-in-Publication Data
Jevon, Philip.
Treating the critically ill patient / Philip Jevon.
p. ; cm. – (Essential clinical skills for nurses)
Includes bibliographical references and index.
ISBN-13: 978-1-4051-4172-7 (pbk. : alk. paper)
1. Critical care nursing. 2. Critical care medicine. I. Title. II. Series.
[DNLM: 1. Critical Illness–therapy. 2. Critical Care–methods. 3. Critical
Illness–nursing. WX 218 J58t 2007]
RT120.I5J48 2007
616.02′8–dc22
2007011917

A catalogue record for this title is available from the British Library

Set in 9/12pt Palatino
by SNP Best-set Typesetter Ltd., Hong Kong
Printed and bound in Singapore
by Utopia Press Pte Ltd

The publisher's policy is to use permanent paper from mills that operate a
sustainable forestry policy, and which has been manufactured from pulp
processed using acid-free and elementary chlorine-free practices.
Furthermore, the publisher ensures that the text paper and cover board
used have met acceptable environmental accreditation standards.

For further information on Blackwell Publishing, visit our website:
www.blackwellnursing.com

Contents

Foreword

The need for timely recognition and treatment of patients who become critically ill has been the recurrent message of research papers and government policy over the past decade. One of the main drivers for this message is the acknowledgement that many of these patients deteriorate outside of critical care units. However, these patients can also often be managed successfully in the acute ward, without the need for transfer to a more intensive level of care. *Treating the Critically Ill Patient* emphasises the steps taken by nurses and other members of the health care team to intervene at an early stage of the patient's worsening condition.

Recent evidence suggests that, when nurses and doctors have patient assessment information at their fingertips, communication of that information (sometimes referred to as the 'art of referral') can be inadequate. Similarly, the development of ICU outreach or medical emergency teams who rescue a 'failing' patient has been noted by some to have a de-skilling effect on ward staff. The contents of this book should serve to empower nurses to communicate patient needs and maintain an active role in the treatment of the deteriorating patient.

The inclusion in this book of chapters on ethics and record keeping reflect two further dimensions of communication when managing critically ill patients. First, we must ensure that adequate communication takes place between patients/family and professionals to ensure that everyone is aware of the patients wishes. Second, written communication should be of the highest possible standard to ensure patients receive optimal care in a timely manner; the importance of nursing records in communicating trends in patient observations cannot be overstated.

I commend this book to all who are involved in the treatment of critically ill patients; it provides both a quick reference in an emergency situation and a sound evidence base for more 'reflective' reading.

Professor Ruth Endacott
Professor of Critical Care Nursing
University of Plymouth, UK
and
La Trobe University, Australia

Acknowledgements

I would like to thank Steve Webb, Becky Mcbride and Ng Yi-Yang for their help with the photographs. I would like to thank Jacko Jackson for giving permission to use this image on the front cover.

Thanks also goes to Dr Pooni who wrote Chapters 7 and 8 and to Tim Simmonds who wrote Chapter 9.

Overview of Treating the Critically Ill Patient

1

INTRODUCTION

Most patients who suffer a cardiopulmonary arrest in hospital will have displayed adverse physiological signs prior to collapse, e.g. tachycardia, tachypnoea, hypotension (Resuscitation Council UK, 2006). The challenge for nurses is to identify 'at risk' patients, for whom deterioration is possible and for whom simple, appropriate and early preventative treatments could prevent deterioration and promote recovery (Smith, 2003). The early recognition of the 'at risk' patient using a 'track and trigger' system is discussed at length in *Monitoring the Critically Ill Patient* (Jevon & Ewens, 2007).

The purpose of this book, however, is to provide a systematic approach to the treatment of the critically ill patient. Prompt recognition and effective early treatment of the critical illness will help to prevent deterioration of the patient and maximize the chances of recovery (Gwinnutt, 2006). The nurse must be able to recognize that the patient is critically ill and, while senior help is on the way, begin effective treatment, within her own sphere of competence. Simple measures, e.g. delivery of high concentration of oxygen, may be all that are required.

The aim of this chapter is to provide an overview of treating the critically ill patient. Subsequent chapters will then systematically discuss the treatment of the critically ill patient.

LEARNING OBJECTIVES

At the end of the chapter the reader will be able to:

- ❏ Discuss what emergency equipment should be available.
- ❏ Describe the assessment and recognition of critical illness.
- ❏ State the aim of treating the critically ill patient.

1

EMERGENCY EQUIPMENT

Wherever critically ill patients are treated, procedures should be in place to ensure that all the essential monitoring and emergency equipment, emergency drugs/fluids are immediately available, accessible and in good working order (Jevon, 2001).

Oxygen

Facilities should be available for the delivery of high concentrations of oxygen. Piped oxygen to a wall outlet behind the patient's bed is ideal. Otherwise a portable oxygen cylinder, fitted with a variable oxygen flow rate meter (Figure 1.1) that can deliver up to 15 l/min, should be immediately available. There should also

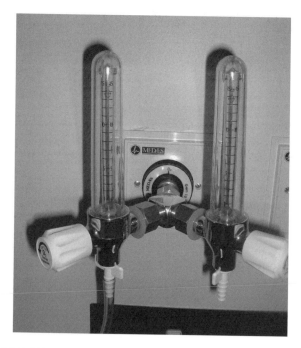

Fig 1.1 Variable rate oxygen flow meter

be adequate stocks of various oxygen delivery devices, particularly non-rebreathe masks (see p. 53).

Suction

Every clinical area should have access to a portable suction device. In addition, it is preferable if 'wall mounted suction' is available behind each patient's bed (Figure 1.2). As suction is sometimes immediately required in a life-threatening situation, it is standard practice to store appropriate suction connection tubing, together with suction catheters (rigid and flexible), with the suction source, i.e. it should be for quick set-up and use.

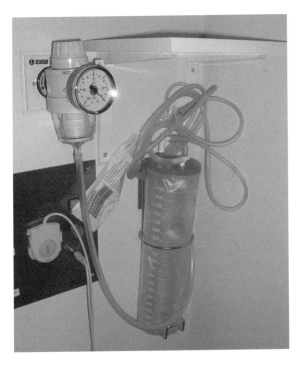

Fig 1.2 Wall mounted suction

Monitoring devices

At the very least, an ECG monitor and a pulse oximeter should be available. Other monitoring facilities e.g. capnography, may also be required in some clinical areas.

Cardiopulmonary resuscitation trolley

A carefully set out and fully stocked cardiac arrest trolley is paramount, following Resuscitation Council (UK) guidelines (Box 1.1)

Box 1.1 Cardiopulmonary resuscitation equipment which should be available (Resuscitation Council UK, 2004a)

Airway equipment

- Pocket mask with oxygen port (should be widely available in all clinical areas)
- Self-inflating resuscitation bag with oxygen reservoir and tubing (ideally, the resuscitation bag should be single use – if not, it should be equipped with a suitable filter)
- Clear face masks, sizes 3, 4 and 5
- Oropharyngeal airways, sizes 2, 3 and 4
- Nasopharyngeal airways, sizes 6 and 7
- Portable suction equipment
- Yankauer suckers
- Tracheal suction catheters, sizes 12 and 14
- Laryngeal mask airways (sizes 4 and 5), or ProSeal LMAs (sizes 4 and 5), or Combitube (small)
- Magill forceps
- Tracheal tubes – oral, cuffed, sizes 6, 7 and 8
- Gum elastic bougie or equivalent device
- Lubricating jelly
- Laryngoscope handles (×2) and blades (standard and long blade)
- Spare batteries for laryngoscope and spare bulbs (if applicable)
- Fixation for tracheal tube (e.g. ribbon gauze/tape)
- Scissors

- Selection of syringes
- Oxygen mask with reservoir (non-rebreathing) bag
- Oxygen cylinders
- Cylinder key

Circulation equipment

- Defibrillator (shock advisory module and/or external pacing facility to be decided by local policy)
- ECG electrodes
- Defibrillation gel pads or self-adhesive defibrillator pads (preferred)
- Selection of intravenous cannulae
- Selection of syringes and needles
- Cannula fixing dressings and tapes
- Seldinger central venous catheter kit
- Intravenous infusion sets
- 0.9% sodium chloride – 1000 ml × 2
- Arterial blood gas syringes
- Tourniquet

Drugs

(a) Immediately available prefilled syringes:

- Adrenaline (epinephrine) 1 mg (1 : 10 000) × 4
- Atropine 3 mg × 1
- Amiodarone 300 mg × 1

(b) Other readily available drugs

Intravenous medications:

- Adenosine 6 mg × 10
- Adrenaline 1 mg (1 : 10 000) × 4
- Adrenaline 1 mg (1 : 1000) × 2
- Amiodarone 300 mg × 1
- Calcium chloride 10 ml of 100 mg/ml × 1
- Chlorphenamine 10 mg × 2
- Furosemide 50 mg × 2

Continued

- Glucose 10% 500 ml × 1
- Hydrocortisone 100 mg × 2
- Lidocaine 100 mg × 1
- Magnesium sulphate 50% solution 2 g (4 ml) × 1
- Midazolam 10 mg × 1
- Naloxone 400 mg × 5
- Normal saline 10-ml ampoules
- Potassium chloride for injection (see *NPSA Alert*)
- Sodium bicarbonate 8.4% – 50 ml × 1

Other medications/equipment:

- Salbutamol (5 mg × 2) and ipratropium bromide (500 mg × 2) nebules
- Nebulizer device and mask
- GTN spray
- Aspirin 300 mg

Additional Items

- Clock
- Gloves/goggles/aprons
- Audit forms
- Sharps container and clinical waste bag
- Large scissors
- Alcohol wipes
- Blood sample bottles
- A sliding sheet or similar device should be available for safer handling

(Resuscitation Council UK, 2004a). The trolley should be spacious, sturdy, easily accessible and mobile; ideally, each trolley in a healthcare establishment should be identically stocked to avoid confusion. A defibrillator should be immediately available and where appropriate, e.g. general wards, it should have an automatic or advisory facility (Jevon, 2001). Defibrillators with external pacing should be strategically located, e.g. A&E, ICU, CCU.

Routine checking of emergency equipment

Emergency equipment should be routinely checked following local protocols. It is recommended that cardiopulmonary resuscitation equipment should be checked on a daily basis by each ward or department responsible for it (Resuscitation Council (UK), 2001b). A system for daily documented checks of the equipment inventory should be in place (Jevon, 2001). The electronic equipment should be stored, maintained and checked following the manufacturer's recommendations and the local Electro Biomedical Engineers Department (EBME).

ASSESSMENT AND RECOGNITION OF CRITICAL ILLNESS

Safety precautions

When approaching the critically ill patient, ensure the environment is safe and free of hazards and follow infection control guidelines, e.g. wash hands, put on gloves if necessary.

Communication with the patient

Talk to the patient and evaluate his response: a normal response indicates he has a clear airway, is breathing and has adequate cerebral perfusion; the inability to complete sentences could indicate extreme respiratory distress. An inappropriate response or no response could indicate an acute life-threatening physiological disturbance (Gwinnutt, 2006).

General appearance of the patient

Note the patient's general appearance, his colour and whether he appears content and relaxed or distressed and anxious.

Senior help

During the assessment process, consider whether senior help should be requested.

Oxygen and patient monitoring devices

Administer high-concentration oxygen, together with appropriate monitoring devices, e.g. pulse oximetry, ECG monitor and non-invasive blood pressure monitoring, as soon as it is safe to do so (Resuscitation Council UK, 2006).

ABCDE assessment

The Resuscitation Council (UK) (2006) has issued guidelines on the recognition and treatment of the critically ill patient. Adapted from the ALERT course (Smith, 2003), these guidelines follow the logical and systematic ABCDE approach to patient assessment:

- **A**irway
- **B**reathing
- **C**irculation
- **D**isability
- **E**xposure

When assessing the patient, undertake a complete initial assessment, identifying and treating life-threatening problems first, before moving on to the next part of the assessment. The effectiveness of treatment/intervention should be evaluated and regular re-assessment undertaken. The need to alert more senior help should be recognized and other members of the multidisciplinary team should be utilized as appropriate so that patient assessment, instigation of appropriate monitoring and interventions can be undertaken simultaneously.

Irrespective of their training, experience and expertise in clinical assessment and treatment, all nurses can follow the ABCDE approach; clinical skills, knowledge, expertise and local circumstances will determine what aspects of the assessment and treatment are undertaken.

Assessment of airway

Look, listen and feel for the signs of airway obstruction. Partial airway obstruction will result in noisy breathing:

- *Gurgling*: indicates the presence of fluid, e.g. secretions or vomit, in the mouth or upper airway; usually seen in a patient with altered consciousness level who is having difficulty or is unable to clear his own airway.
- *Snoring*: indicates that the pharynx is being partially obstructed by the tongue; usually seen in a patient with altered consciousness level lying in a supine position.
- *Stridor*: high-pitched sound during inspiration, indicating partial upper airway obstruction; usually due to either a foreign body or laryngeal oedema.
- *Wheeze*: noisy musical whistling type sound due to the turbulent flow of air through narrowed bronchi and bronchioles, more pronounced on expiration; causes include asthma and chronic obstructive pulmonary disorder (COPD).

Complete airway obstruction can be detected by lack of air movement at the patient's mouth and nose. Paradoxical chest and abdominal movements ('see-saw' movement of the chest) may be observed and, if not rapidly treated, central cyanosis will develop (late sign of airway obstruction).

'Treat airway obstruction as a medical emergency and obtain expert help immediately. Untreated, airway obstruction leads to a lowered PaO_2 and risks hypoxic damage to the brain, kidneys and heart, cardiac arrest, and even death' (Resuscitation Council UK, 2005). Treating airway obstruction is discussed in Chapter 2.

Assessment of breathing

Look, listen and feel to assess breathing:

Count the respiratory rate: normal respiratory rate is 12–20/min (Resuscitation Council UK, 2006). Tachypnoea is usually the first sign that the patient has respiratory distress (Smith, 2003). Bradypnoea is an ominous sign and could indicate imminent respiratory arrest; causes include drugs, e.g. opiates, fatigue, hypothermia, head injury and CNS depression.

Evaluate chest movement: chest movement should be symmetrical; unilateral chest movement suggests unilateral pathology e.g. pneumothorax, pneumonia, pleural effusion (Smith, 2003).

Evaluate depth of breathing: only marked degrees of hyperventilation and hypoventilation can be detected; hyperventilation may be seen in metabolic acidosis or anxiety and hypoventilation may be seen in opiate toxicity (Ford *et al.*, 2005).

Evaluate respiratory pattern: Cheyne-Stokes breathing pattern (periods of apnoea alternating with periods of hyperpnoea) can be associated with brain stem ischaemia, cerebral injury and severe left ventricular failure (altered carbon dioxide sensitivity of the respiratory centre) (Ford *et al.*, 2005).

Note the oxygen saturation (SaO$_2$) reading: normal is 97–100%. A low SaO$_2$ could indicate respiratory distress or compromise. NB the pulse oximeter does not detect hypercapnia and the SaO$_2$ can be normal in the presence of a very high PaCO$_2$ (Resuscitation Council UK, 2006).

Listen to the breathing: normal breathing is quiet. Rattling airway noises indicate the presence of airway secretions, usually due to the patient being unable to cough sufficiently or unable to take a deep breath in (Smith, 2003). The presence of stridor or wheeze indicates partial, but significant, airway obstruction (see above).

Check the position of the trachea: place the tip of the index finger into the supersternal notch, let it slip either side of the trachea and determine whether it fits more easily into one or other side of the trachea (Ford *et al.*, 2005). Deviation of the trachea to one side indicates mediastinal shift (e.g. pneumothorax, lung fibrosis or pleural fluid).

- *Palpate the chest wall*: to detect surgical emphysema or crepitus (suggesting a pneumothorax *until* proven otherwise) (Smith, 2003).
- *Perform chest percussion*: place the left hand on the patient's chest wall. Ensure the fingers are slightly separated, with the middle finger pressed firmly into the intercostal space to be percussed (Ford *et al.*, 2005).

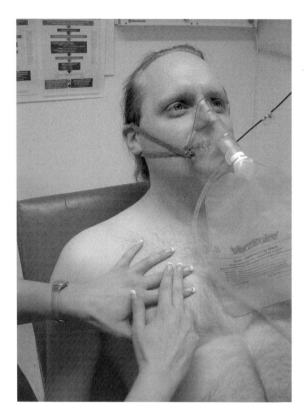

Fig 1.3 Chest percussion

- Strike the centre of the middle phalanx of the middle finger sharply using the tip of the middle finger of the right hand (Ford *et al.*, 2005) (Figure 1.3). Deliver the stroke using a quick flick of the wrist and finger joints, not from the arm or shoulder. The percussing finger should be bent so that the terminal phalanx is at right angles to the metacarpal bones when the blow is delivered, and it strikes the percussed finger in a per-pendicular way. The percussing finger should then be removed immediately, like a clapper inside a bell, otherwise the resultant sound will be dampened (Epstein *et al.*, 2003).

- Percuss the anterior and lateral chest wall. Percuss from side to side, top to bottom, comparing both sides and looking for asymmetry.
- Categorize the percussion sounds (see below).
- If an area of altered resonance is located, map out its boundaries by percussing from areas of normal to altered resonance (Ford *et al.*, 2005).
- Sit the patient forward and then percuss the posterior chest wall, omitting the areas covered by the scapulae. Ask the patient to move his elbows forward across the front of his chest: this will rotate the scapulae anteriorly and out of the way (Talley & O'Connor, 2001). It may be helpful to offer the patient a pillow to lean on.
- Again percuss from side to side, top to bottom, comparing both sides and looking for asymmetry. Don't forget that the lung extends much further down posteriorly than anteriorly (Epstein *et al.*, 2004).
- Categorize the percussion sounds (see below).

Causes of different percussion notes:

- *Resonant*: air-filled lung
- *Dull*: liver, spleen, heart, lung consolidation/collapse
- *Stoney dull*: pleural effusion/thickening
- *Hyper-resonant*: pneumothorax, emphysema
- *Tympanitic*: gas-filled viscus.

(Source: Ford *et al.*, 2005)

Auscultate the chest (Figure 1.4):

- Ask the patient to breath in and out normally through his mouth.
- Auscultate the anterior chest from side to side, and top to bottom. Auscultate over equivalent areas and compare the volume and character of the sounds and note any additional sounds. Compare the sounds during inspiration and expiration.

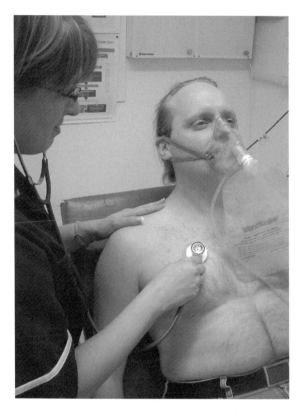

Fig 1.4 Chest auscultation

- Note the location and quality of the sounds heard.
- Auscultate the posterior chest, from side to side, and top to bottom. Auscultate over equivalent areas and compare the volume and character of the sounds and note any additional sounds. Compare the sounds during inspiration and expiration.

(Jevon, 2006)

Evaluate air entry, the depth of breathing and the equality of breath sounds on both sides of the chest. Bronchial breathing indicates lung consolidation; absent or reduced sounds suggest a pneumothorax or pleural fluid (Smith, 2003). In particular, note any additional breath sounds:

- *Wheezes (rhonchi)*: high-pitched musical sounds associated with air being forced through narrowed airways, e.g. asthma (Ford *et al.*, 2005). Usually more pronounced on expiration. Inspiratory wheeze (stridor) is usually indicative of severe upper airway obstruction, e.g. foreign body, laryngeal oedema. If both inspiratory and expiratory wheezes heard, this is usually due to excessive airway secretions (Adam & Osborne, 2005).
- *Crackles (crepitations)*: non-musical sounds – associated with reopening of collapsed airway, e.g. pulmonary oedema (Ford *et al.*, 2005). Crackles are usually localized in pneumonia and mild cases of bronchiectasis; in pulmonary oedema and fibrosing alveolitis, both lung bases are equally affected (Epstein *et al.*, 2003).
- *Pleural friction rub*: leathery/creaking sounds during inspiration and expiration, evident in areas of inflammation when the normally smooth pleural surfaces are roughened and rub on each other (Adam & Osborne, 2005).

Record peak expiratory flow rate: provides a useful estimate of the calibre of the airways particularly in asthma and chronic obstructive pulmonary disease (Ford *et al.*, 2005).

Evaluate efficacy of breathing, work of breathing and adequacy of ventilation:

- Efficacy of breathing: air entry, chest movement, pulse oximetry
- Arterial blood gas analysis and capnography
- Work of breathing: respiratory rate and accessory muscle use, e.g. neck and abdominal muscles
- Adequacy of ventilation: heart rate, skin colour and mental status.

If the patient has compromised breathing it is paramount to provide prompt effective treatment. In addition, during the initial assessment of breathing, it is essential to diagnose and effectively treat immediately life-threatening conditions, e.g. acute severe asthma, pulmonary oedema, tension pneumothorax, massive haemothorax (Resuscitation Council UK, 2006). The treatment of compromised breathing is discussed in Chapter 3.

Assessment of circulation

Look, listen and feel to assess circulation.

Palpate peripheral and central pulses: presence, rate, quality, regularity and equality (Smith, 2003). A weak thready pulse suggests a poor cardiac output and bounding pulse may indicate sepsis (Resuscitation Council UK, 2006).

Check the colour and temperature of the hands and fingers: signs of cardiovascular compromise include cool and pale peripheries.

Measure the capillary refill time (CRT): apply sufficient pressure to cause blanching to the skin, e.g. sternum, for 5 s and then release (Figure 1.5). Normal CRT is < 2 s; a prolonged CRT could indicate poor peripheral perfusion, although other causes can include cool ambient temperature, poor lighting and old age (Resuscitation Council UK, 2006).

Look for other signs of a poor cardiac output: e.g. altered consciousness level and, if the patient has a urinary catheter, oliguria (urine volume < 0.5 ml/kg per hour) (Smith, 2003).

Look for signs of haemorrhage: e.g. from wounds or drains, or evidence of internal haemorrhage, e.g. abdominal swelling; concealed blood loss can be significant, even if drains are empty (Smith, 2003).

Measure blood pressure: systolic BP < 90 mmHg suggests shock. Normal blood pressure does not exclude shock because compensatory mechanisms increase peripheral resistance in response to reduced cardiac output (Smith, 2003). A low diastolic BP suggests arterial vasodilation, e.g. anaphylaxis or

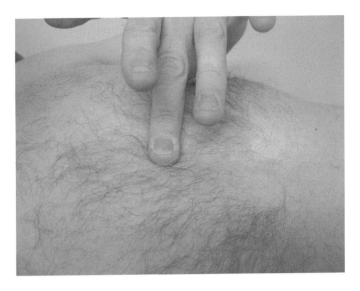

Fig 1.5 Measuring capillary refill time

sepsis. A narrowed pulse pressure, i.e. the difference between systolic and diastolic readings (normal is 35–45 mmHg), suggests arterial vasoconstriction, e.g. cardiogenic shock or hypovolaemia (Resuscitation Council UK, 2006).

Assess the state of the veins: if hypovolaemia is present the veins could be under-filled or collapsed (Smith, 2003).

Interpret the ECG: determine whether a cardiac arrhythmia is present. A 12-lead ECG should be recorded as a priority in some situations, e.g. chest pain.

In almost all medical and surgical emergencies, if the patient is hypotensive, hypovolaemia should be considered to be the primary cause of shock, until proven otherwise (Resuscitation Council UK, 2006). The treatment of hypotension is discussed in Chapter 4. The treatment of a patient with a bradycardia or tachycardia is discussed in Chapter 5. The treatment of oliguria is discussed in Chapter 7.

Box 1.2 AVPU scale

Alert
Responds to **v**oice
Responds to **p**ain
Unconscious
(Resuscitation Council UK, 2006)

Assessment of disability

Assess disability (central nervous system function).

Evaluate the patient's level of consciousness: use AVPU (Box 1.2) or the Glasgow Coma Scale (GCS) if a more objective assessment of consciousness level is required, e.g. head injury (see Chapter 6).

Examine the pupils: compare size, equality and reaction to light of each pupil.

Undertake bedside glucose measurement: exclude hypoglycaemia as a cause of altered consciousness level.

The treatment of a patient with altered consciousness level is discussed in Chapter 6.

Exposure

Expose the patient and undertake a thorough examination to ensure important details are not overlooked (Smith, 2003). In particular, the examination should concentrate on the part of the body which is most likely to be contributing to the patient's ill status, e.g. in suspected anaphylaxis, examine the skin for urticaria. Respect the patient's dignity and minimize heat loss. In addition:

- Take a full clinical history and review the patient's notes/charts
- Study the recorded vital signs: trends are more significant than one-off recordings
- Administer prescribed medications

- Review laboratory results and ECG and radiological investigations
- Ascertain what level of care the patient requires (e.g. ward, HDU, ICU)
- Document in the patient's notes details of assessment, treatment and response to treatment.

(Source: Resuscitation Council UK, 2006)

Treatment of a patient with oliguria, abnormal temperature and pain is discussed in Chapters 7, 8 and 9.

AIM OF TREATING THE CRITICALLY ILL PATIENT

The aim of treating the critical ill patient is the early anticipation and detection of abnormal physiology at a stage before organ failure is established and to initiate simple preventative therapies and interventions (Smith, 2003). The treatment should be seen as a 'holding measure' to keep the patient alive and to produce some clinical improvement, in order that definitive treatment may be initiated (Resuscitation Council UK, 2005).

CONCLUSION

Recognition and effective treatment of the acutely ill patient is paramount. In this chapter the importance of ensuring that the necessary emergency equipment is available and the assessment and recognition of the critically ill patient following the ABCDE approach have been described. In the remaining chapters the specific treatment for the critically ill patient will be discussed.

REFERENCES

Adam, S, & Osborne, S. (2005) *Critical Care Nursing Science and Practice*, 2nd edn. Oxford University Press, Oxford.

Epstein, O, Perkin, G, Cookson, J, de Bono, D. (2003) *Clinical Examination*, 3rd edn. Mosby, London.

Ford, M, Hennessey, I, Japp, A. (2005) *Introduction to Clinical Examination.* Elsevier, Oxford.

Gwinnutt, C. (2006) *Clinical Anaesthesia,* 2nd edn. Blackwell Publishing, Oxford.

Jevon, P. (2001) *Advanced Cardiac Life Support.* Butterworth Heinemann, Oxford.

Jevon, P, & Ewens, B. (2007) *Monitoring the Critically Ill Patient,* 2nd edn. Blackwell Publishing, Oxford.

Resuscitation Council (UK) (2004a) *Recommended Minimum Equipment for In-Hospital Adult Resuscitation.* Resuscitation Council (UK), London.

Resuscitation Council (UK) (2004b) *Cardiopulmonary Resuscitation*: *Standards for Clinical Practice and Training: a joint statement from Royal College of Anaesthetists, Royal College of Physicians of London, Intensive Care Society and Resuscitation Council (UK).* Resuscitation Council UK, London.

Resuscitation Council (UK) (2005) *Guidelines 2005.* Resuscitation Council (UK), London.

Resuscitation Council (UK) (2006) *Advanced Life Support,* 5th edn. Resuscitation Council UK, London.

Smith, G. (2003) *ALERT Acute Life-Threatening Events Recognition and Treatment,* 2nd edn. University of Portsmouth, Portsmouth.

Talley, N, & O'Connor, S. (2001) *Clinical Examination,* 4th edn. Blackwell Publishing, Oxford.

2 Treating a Patient with Airway Obstruction

INTRODUCTION

Airway obstruction can be life threatening; it can be partial or complete and can occur at any level of the respiratory tract from the mouth to the trachea (Smith, 2003). If untreated, it can lead to hypoxaemia, resulting in hypoxic damage to the brain, kidneys and heart; cardiac arrest and even death may ensue (Resuscitation Council UK, 2006).

Airway obstruction can be subtle and is often undetected by healthcare professionals (Nolan *et al.*, 2005). Recognition of airway obstruction can be achieved by following the familiar look, listen and feel technique (see Chapter 1). Once airway obstruction has been recognized, immediate action should be taken to relieve the obstruction (Resuscitation Council UK, 2006). Basic airway opening manoeuvres can usually relieve the obstruction; simple airway adjuncts may also be required (Gwinnutt, 2006). Sometimes advanced airway intervention, e.g. tracheal intubation, will be necessary. The priority is to recognize airway obstruction, call for help and take appropriate remedial action.

The aim of this chapter is to understand the treatment of a patient with airway obstruction.

LEARNING OBJECTIVES

At the end of this chapter the reader will be able to:

❑ List the causes of airway obstruction
❑ Discuss the signs of airway obstruction
❑ Describe the principles of airway management
❑ Outline the treatment of airway obstruction.

CAUSES OF AIRWAY OBSTRUCTION

Causes of airway obstruction include:

- *Tongue*: this is the commonest cause of airway obstruction in a semiconscious or unconscious patient – relaxation of the muscles supporting the tongue can result in it falling back and blocking the pharynx
- *Vomit, blood and secretions*
- *Foreign body*
- *Tissue swelling*: causes include anaphylaxis, trauma or infection
- *Laryngeal oedema*: due to burns, inflammation or allergy occurring at the level of the larynx
- *Laryngeal spasm*: due to foreign body, airway stimulation or secretions/blood in the airway
- *Tracheobronchial obstruction*: due to aspiration of gastric contents, secretions, pulmonary oedema fluid or bronchospasm.

(Sources: Smith, 2003 and Gwinnutt, 2006)

SIGNS OF AIRWAY OBSTRUCTION

If the patient is talking he has a patent airway. In complete airway obstruction, there are no breath sounds at the mouth or nose. Paradoxical chest and abdominal movements ('see-saw' respirations) and the use of the accessory muscles of respiration may be evident. Central cyanosis is a late sign of airway obstruction.

In partial airway obstruction, air entry is diminished and often noisy. Certain noises will assist in localizing the level of the obstruction (Smith, 2003):

- *Gurgling*: fluid in the mouth or upper airway
- *Snoring*: tongue partially obstructing the pharynx
- *Crowing*: laryngeal spasm
- *Inspiratory stridor*: 'croaking respirations' indicating partial upper airway obstruction, e.g. foreign body, laryngeal oedema
- *Expiratory wheeze*: noisy musical sound caused by turbulent flow of air through narrowed bronchi and bronchioles, more pronounced on expiration; causes include asthma and chronic obstructive airways disorder.

PRINCIPLES OF AIRWAY MANAGEMENT

Airway obstruction is an emergency and can be life threatening. All nurses should understand the principles of basic airway management, as basic techniques are usually all that are required to open and clear the patient's airway. In this section, the principles of basic airway management will be discussed. For the reader's information, an overview of the principles of advanced airway management is provided in Appendix 1 and Appendix 2.

Head tilt and chin lift

Head tilt and chin lift can improve airway patency when the tongue or other upper airway structures, e.g. soft palate and epiglottis, are the cause of the obstruction (Nolan *et al.*, 2005). It can achieve airway patency in 91% of cases (Guildner, 1976), by stretching the anterior tissues of the neck and displacing the tongue forward away from the posterior pharyngeal wall and lifting the epiglottis from the laryngeal opening (Safar, 1958). A pillow under the patient's head and shoulders can help to maintain this position (Jevon, 2006). To perform head tilt and chin lift:

- Place the one hand on the patient's forehead and gently tilt the head back; at the same time place the fingertips of the other hand under the point of the patient's chin and lift the chin upwards (Figure 2.1) (Jevon, 2006).

Jaw thrust

In the jaw thrust manoeuvre (Figure 2.2) the mandible is displaced anteriorly (together with the tongue) using the index fingers positioned just proximal to the angles of the jaw. At the same time, pressure by the thumbs on the chin can help to open the mouth.

Use the jaw thrust if the patient has a suspected cervical spine injury to establish a clear upper airway (Nolan *et al.*, 2005), as head tilt may aggravate the injury and damage the spinal cord.

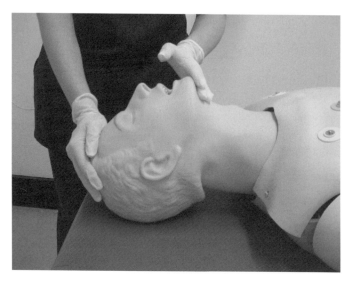

Fig 2.1 Head tilt and chin lift

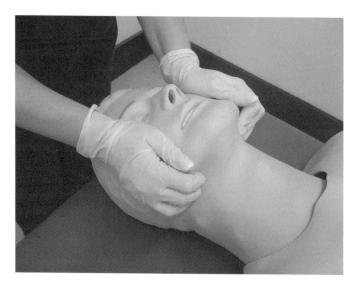

Fig 2.2 Jaw thrust manoeuvre

This should be accompanied by manual in-line immobilization of the head and neck by an assistant (Nolan & Parr, 1997).

If life-threatening airway obstruction persists, despite the application of effective jaw thrust or chin lift, head tilt should be performed gradually more and more until airway patency is achieved: the establishment of a clear airway takes priority over concerns about potential injury to the cervical spine (Nolan *et al.*, 2005).

Re-assess (look, listen and feel) to ensure that an open and clear airway has been achieved and continually monitor its continued patency.

Suction

If vomit/fluid/blood is present in the airway, turn the patient's head on the side and apply suction using a wide-bore rigid (Yankeur) catheter (Figure 2.3a). This device can provide rapid suction of large volumes of vomit, secretions, etc., from the mouth and pharynx (Jevon, 2006). Use a flexible suction catheter (Figure 2.3b) if applying suction down an airway adjunct, e.g. oropharyngeal airway or a tracheal tube. If there is a foreign body in the mouth, remove it using a pair of Magills forceps (Figure 2.4).

To minimize deoxygenation, suction should not be applied for longer than 10s (Idris *et al.*, 1996). If the patient has an intact gag reflex, the suction catheter should be used with caution because it could induce vomiting (Resuscitation Council UK, 2006).

Suction should be immediately available for all patients who are at risk of aspiration, e.g. unconscious patients (Jevon, 2006). Wall-mounted suction behind the bed is preferable; a portable suction device will be required if the patient is being transferred (Jevon, 2006).

Oropharyngeal and nasopharyngeal airways

The oropharyngeal (Guedel) and nasopharyngeal airways can provide an artificial passage for airflow by separating the posterior pharyngeal wall from the tongue, although the position of the patient's head and neck must also be maintained in order to

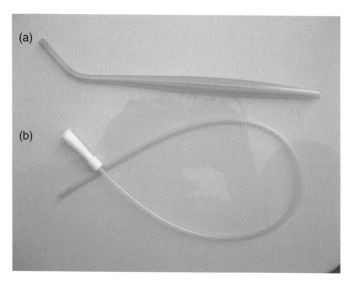

Fig 2.3a Wide-bore rigid (Yankeur) catheter
Fig 2.3b Flexible suction catheter

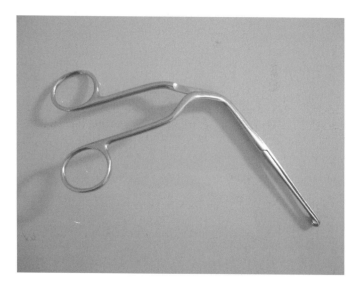

Fig 2.4 Magill's forceps

keep the airway aligned and simultaneous head tilt and jaw thrust may also be required (Nolan *et al.*, 2005). The use of a nasopharyngeal airway may be helpful in situations when oropharyngeal airway insertion is difficult, e.g. patient with clenched teeth (Smith, 2003).

An oropharyngeal airway (Figure 2.5) is a curved plastic tube, flattened in cross section with a flange (projecting flat rim) at the oral end. It is designed to lie over the tongue, preventing it from falling back into the pharynx. Available in a variety of sizes, an appropriately sized oropharyngeal airway is one that holds the tongue in the normal anatomical position, following its natural curvature (Idris *et al.*, 1996). If it is too big, it could occlude the patient's airway by displacing the epiglottis, could hinder the use of a face mask and could damage laryngeal structures; if it is too small, it could occlude the airway by pushing the tongue back

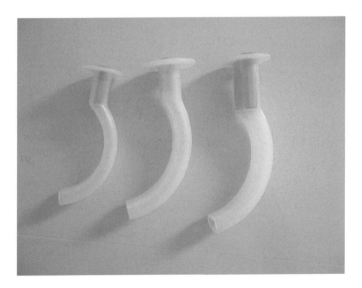

Fig 2.5 Oropharyngeal airway

(Jevon, 2006). In small, medium and large adults airway sizes 2, 3 and 4 respectively, are used (Nolan *et al.*, 2005).

Following the correct insertion technique will help to minimize the risk of unnecessary trauma to the delicate tissues in the mouth and to avoid inadvertently blocking the patient's airway (Jevon, 2006). The oropharyngeal airway should be used only if the patient is unconscious because, if glossopharyngeal and laryngeal reflexes are present, it could induce vomiting and laryngospasm (Mehta, 1990).

The following procedure is recommended for inserting an oropharyngeal airway:

- If necessary, suction the patient's airway.
- Estimate the correct size by comparing the length of the airway with the vertical distance from the patient's incisors and the angle of the jaw (Figure 2.6) (Gwinnutt, 2006). Oropharyngeal

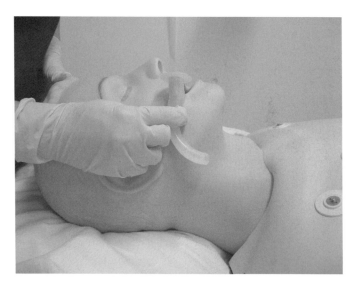

Fig 2.6 Oropharyngeal airway: estimate the correct size by comparing the length of the airway to the vertical distance from the patient's incisors and the angle of the jaw

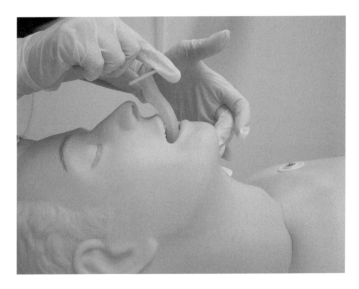

Fig 2.7 Oropharyngeal airway insertion: open the patient's mouth and insert the airway upside down as far as the hard palate

airway sizes 2, 3 and 4 are normally adequate for small, medium and large adults, respectively (Nolan *et al.*, 2005).

- If possible, lubricate the airway before insertion.
- Open the patient's mouth and insert the airway upside down as far as the hard palate in the inverted position (Figure 2.7) (the curved part of the airway will help depress the tongue downwards, preventing it from being pushed posteriorly) (Jevon, 2006).
- As the airway passes over the soft palate, rotate the airway through 180° and continue inserting until the flange lies in front of the teeth, or gums if the patient is edentulous.
- Following insertion, re-assess to confirm the airway is patent.
- Closely monitor the patency and position of the airway; it can become blocked by the tongue or epiglottis and can become wedged into the vallecula (Marsh *et al.*, 1991). Vomit, secretions

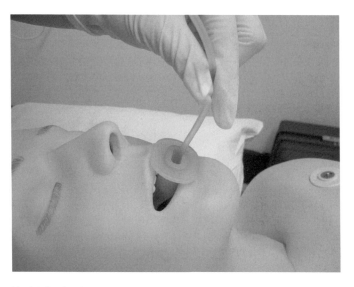

Fig 2.8 Suction down an oropharyngeal airway

and blood can also compromise its patency; if suction down the airway tube is required, use a flexible correctly sized catheter (Figure 2.8).

The nasopharyngeal airway (Figure 2.9) is a flexible, soft plastic tube with a flange at the nasal end and a bevelled edge at the pharyngeal end. As it is less likely to induce gagging than an oropharyngeal airway, it can be used in a semiconscious or conscious patient when the airway is at risk of being compromised (Jevon, 2002). It can be life saving in a patient with a clenched jaw, trismus or maxillofacial injuries (Jevon, 2006).

The use of a nasopharyngeal airway has been previously contraindicated in patients with a suspected base of skull fracture, as it could penetrate the cranial fossa (Muzzi *et al.*, 1991). However, although an oropharyngeal airway is preferred in these patients, if it is not possible to insert it and the airway is obstructed, careful

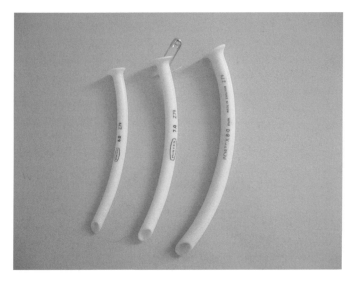

Fig 2.9 Nasopharyngeal airways

insertion of a nasopharyngeal airway could be life saving, i.e. the benefits may far outweigh the risks (Nolan *et al.*, 2005).

A correctly sized airway should be used: if it is too short it will be ineffective and if it is too long it may enter the oesophagus, causing distension and hypoventilation, or may stimulate the laryngeal or glossopharyngeal reflexes, causing laryngospasm and vomiting (Resuscitation Council UK, 2000). The airways are sized on their internal diameter in millimetres; the larger the diameter, the longer the length.

Traditionally, it has been recommended to measure the diameter against the patient's little finger or anterior nares to determine the correct sized nasopharyngeal airway to use (Nolan *et al.*, 2005). However, these two methods are unreliable, because they do not correlate well with the patient's airway anatomy (Roberts & Porter, 2003). In adults, sizes 7–8 are used (Nolan *et al.*, 2005).

The following procedure is recommended for insertion of a nasopharyngeal airway:

- Select an appropriately sized airway. Sizes 6–7 are suitable for adults (Nolan *et al.*, 2005). As a precaution to prevent inhalation of the airway, some devices require a safety pin to be inserted through the flange.
- Check the patency of the right nostril and lubricate the airway using water-soluble jelly.
- Insert the airway into the nostril, with the bevel facing medially to avoid catching the turbinate bones in the nasal cavity.
- Pass the airway vertically along the floor of the nose, using a slight twisting action, into the posterior pharynx (Figure 2.10) (Resuscitation Council UK, 2006). If there is resistance, remove the airway and try the left nostril (Jevon, 2006). Force should

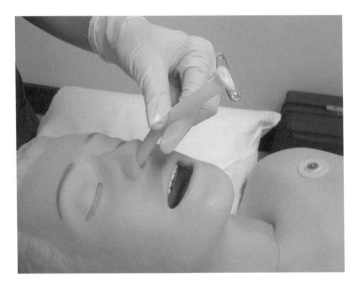

Fig 2.10 Insertion of nasopharyngeal airway: pass the airway vertically along the floor of the nose, using a slight twisting action, into the posterior pharynx

not be used as this could provoke severe bleeding (Gwinnutt, 2006). Once the airway is inserted, the flange should be at the level of the nostril.

- Secure the airway with tape.
- Regularly reassess the patency of the airway.

The recovery position

If the patient is unconscious, the airway could be compromised by regurgitated gastric contents, debris in the mouth or upper airway, loose dentures or mechanical obstruction arising from structures in the mouth, e.g. the tongue and epiglottis (Quinn, 1998). Steps should be taken to protect the airway and prevent further complications, e.g. aspiration of gastric contents: the patient may need to be nursed on his side or with the head end of the bed tilted up (Resuscitation Council UK, 2006).

The recovery position is designed to maintain a patent airway and reduce the risk of airway obstruction and aspiration (American Heart Association, 2005). Placing the patient in the recovery position should be considered if the airway is considered to be at risk, e.g. if there is altered consciousness level.

The recovery position is also recommended in many other situations where the patient's consciousness level is compromised, e.g. following a major seizure (Hayes, 2004 and Bingham, 2004) and during a hypoglycaemic coma (Diebel, 1999).

If the patient has a known or suspected spinal injury, he should be moved only if an open airway cannot otherwise be maintained. Ideally, the patient should be kept still in the position in which he is found, while awaiting the arrival of the emergency services. However, if it is necessary to move the patient, e.g. compromised airway, the patient should ideally be carefully log-rolled, with the head and neck kept as still as possible and in alignment. Extension of the lower arm above the head together with bending both legs, while rolling the head onto the arm, may be feasible (American Heart Association, 2005).

Historically the left lateral position has been advocated for the recovery position (Eastwick-Field, 1996). However, there appear to be no cardiac autonomic tone advantages to be gained by placing a person in the recovery position on one side compared with the other (Ryan *et al.*, 2003). The position will be regularly rotated to minimize the risk of the development of pressure sores.

There are several different variations of the recovery position, each with its own advantages (Handley *et al.*, 2005). However, no single technique is perfect for all patients (Turner *et al.*, 1998 and Handley, 1993). The position used should be stable, near a true lateral position with the head dependent and no pressure applied to the chest which could impair breathing (American Heart Association, 2005).

The following procedure for the recovery position has been adapted from Resuscitation Council UK (2006) guidelines. It is important to follow local manual handling policies, request help from colleagues as appropriate and make use of hospital equipment/facilities, e.g. pillows. A suggested procedure for use in a patient on a bed in hospital is:

- Request help from colleagues.
- Ascertain which side the patient needs to be placed onto.
- Ensure the bed is a suitable height.
- Stand beside the patient's bed. To minimize the risk of self-injury, adopt a stable base with the knees a shoulder-width apart, avoid twisting the back and keep the spine in a neutral position (Resuscitation Council UK, 2001).
- Ensure that both of the patient's legs are straight.
- Position the arm nearest to the nurse perpendicular to the patient's body with the elbow bent and the hand palm uppermost.
- Grasp the far arm and bring it across the patient's chest and hold the back of the hand against the patient's cheek.
- Using the free hand, grasp the far leg just above the knee and pull it up, taking care to keep the patient's foot on the ground.
- Whilst holding the patient's hand against his cheek, pull on the far leg to roll the patient towards you onto his side.

- Adjust the patient's upper leg, ensuring that both the hip and the knee are bent at right angles.
- Tilt the patient's head back to ensure that the airway remains open.
- If necessary, adjust the hand under the patient's cheek to maintain the head tilted.
- Make use of pillows to maintain the position.
- Monitor the patient's vital signs.
- Alternate the patient's position following local procedures.

Guidelines from the Resuscitation Council (UK) (2001) on safer handling during resuscitation should be observed to reduce the risk of self-injury:

- Assess the situation
- Adopt a position close to and directly facing the patient
- Avoid twisting the back
- Keep the spine in a neutral position
- Face the patient straight on.

Even if the patient is in the recovery position, airway, breathing and circulation can still become compromised. Closely monitor the patient's vitals signs, particularly breathing (Handley *et al.*, 2005).

It has been reported that when the lower arm is placed in front, compression of vessels and nerves in the dependent limb can occur (Fulstow & Smith, 1993 and Turner *et al.*, 1997). Although the use of well-placed pillows will help to prevent this from occurring, still monitor for signs of impaired blood flow in the lowermost arm (Rathgeber *et al.*, 1996) and ensure that the patient's position is regularly changed. Problem associated immobility, e.g. pressure sores, can also occur.

TREATING THE PATIENT WITH AIRWAY OBSTRUCTION

Treat airway obstruction as a medical emergency and obtain expert help immediately (Resuscitation Council UK, 2006).

- Try to identify the cause of the obstruction and treat accordingly.
- Use simple methods initially, as these are often very effective (Gwinnutt, 2006). Always evaluate the effectiveness of any intervention. Advanced techniques, e.g. tracheal intubation (Appendix 1), may be required, hence the importance of requesting expert help.
- Administer high-concentration oxygen to the patient.
- *Fluid in the airway* (gurgling sounds can usually be heard): place patient in the lateral position and apply suction, usually with a rigid wide-bore catheter. If the patient has an airway 'tube' in place, e.g. tracheostomy tube, apply suction down the tube using a flexible catheter.
- *Tongue blocking the airway* (snoring sounds may be heard): perform head tilt/chin lift or jaw thrust; place the patient in the recovery position; if the patient is unconscious, insert an oropharyngeal airway. If the patient is semi-conscious, it may be helpful to insert a nasopharyngeal airway.
- *Foreign body airway obstruction* (patient may not be able to speak or breathe properly): encourage the patient to cough; if the cough is ineffective, back slaps and abdominal thrusts may be required (see Appendix 2).
- If airway obstruction is secondary to pathology around the upper airway, expert help should be summoned immediately (Gwinnutt, 2006), e.g. a patient having an anaphylactic reaction who is developing stridor – this usually indicates the development of life-threatening laryngeal oedema which could occlude the airway. Expert help, e.g. senior anaesthetist, should be summoned immediately.
- Apply cricoid pressure (Appendix 3) as directed by the anaesthetist, e.g. during induction of anaesthesia.

CONCLUSION

Airway obstruction can be life threatening; if untreated, it can lead to hypoxaemia, resulting in hypoxic damage to the brain, kidneys and heart; cardiac arrest and even death may ensue (Resuscitation Council UK, 2006).

Once recognized, immediate action to relieve the obstruction is paramount. Try simple methods first. This chapter has discussed the treatment of airway obstruction.

REFERENCES

American Heart Association (2005) 2005 American Heart Association Guidelines for Cardiopulmonary Resuscitation and Emergency cardiovascular care. *Circulation* **112,** 24 (Suppl.).

Bingham, E. (2004) Epilepsy: diagnosis and support for people with epilepsy. *Practice Nursing* **15,** 64–70.

Bryant, A. (1999) The use of cricoid pressure during emergency intubation. *J Emergency Nursing* **25,** 283–284.

Cheek, T, & Gutsche, B. (1993) Pulmonary aspiration of gastric contents. In: Shnider, S, & Levinson, G, eds. *Anesthesia for Obstetrics,* 3rd edn. Williams & Wilkins, Baltimore.

Dean, R. (2005) Emergency first aid for nurses. *Nursing Standard* **20,** 57–65,

Diebel, G. (1999) The management of hypoglycaemia in type1 and type 2 diabetes. *Br J Community Nursing* **4,** 454–460.

Eastwick-Field, P. (1996) Resuscitation: basic life support. *Nursing Standard* **10,** 49–56.

Feinstein, R, & Owens, W. (1992) Anesthesia for ear, nose and throat surgery. In: Barash, P, *et al.,* eds. *Clinical Anesthesia,* 2nd edn. Lippincott, Philadelphia.

Fulstow, R, & Smith, G. (1993) The new recovery position, a cautionary tale. *Resuscitation* **26,** 89–91.

Handley, A. (1993) Recovery position. *Resuscitation* **26,** 93–95.

Handley, A, Koster, R, Monsieurs, K, *et al.* (2005) European Resuscitation Council Guidelines for Resuscitation 2005: Section 2. Adult basic life support and use of automated external defibrillators. *Resuscitation* **67S1,** S7–S23.

Hartsilver, E, & Vanner, R. (2000) Airway obstruction with cricoid pressure. *Anaesthesia* **55,** 208–211.

Hayes, C. (2004) Clinical skills: practical guide for managing adults with epilepsy. *Br J Nursing* **13,** 380–387.

Heath, K, Palmer, M, Fletcher, S. (1996) Fracture of cricoid cartilage after Sellick's manoeuvre. *Br J Anaesth* **76,** 877–888.

Jevon, P. (2002) *Advanced Cardiac Life Support.* Butterworth Heinemann, Oxford.

Koziol, C, Cuddeford, J, Moos, D. (2000) Assessing the force generated with application of cricoid pressure. *AORN* **72,** 1018–1030.

Marsh, A, Nunn, J, Taylor, S, Charlesworth, C. (1991) Airway obstruction associated with the use of the Guedel airway. *Br J Anaes* **67,** 517–523.

Mehrotra, D, & Paust, J. (1979) Antacids and cricoid pressure in preventing regurgitation of gastric contents. *Anesthesiology* **32,** 553–555.

Muzzi, D, Losasso, T, Cucchiara, R. (1991) Complication from a nasopharyngeal airway in a patient with a basilar skull fracture. *Anesthesiology* **74,** 366–368.

Nolan, J, Deakin, C, Soar, J *et al.* (2005) European Resuscitation Council Guidelines for Resuscitation 2005: Section 4. Adult advanced life support. *Resuscitation* **675S,** S39–S86.

Parbrook, G, Davis, P, Parbrook, E. (1990) *Basic Physics and Measurement in Anaesthesia,* 3rd edn. Butterworth Heinemann, Oxford.

Quinn, T. (1998) Cardiopulmonary resuscitation: new European guidelines. *Br J Nursing* **7,** 1070–1077.

Rathgeber, J, Panzer, W, Gunther, U *et al.* (1996) Influence of different types of recovery positions on perfusion indices of the forearm. *Resuscitation* **32,** 13–17.

Resuscitation Council (UK) (2005) *Guidelines 2005.* Resuscitation Council (UK), London.

Resuscitation Council (UK) (2006) *Advanced Life Support Provider Manual,* 5th edn. Resuscitation Council (UK), London.

Resuscitation Council (UK) (2001) *Guidance for Safer Handling During Resuscitation in Hospitals.* Resuscitation Council (UK), London.

Roberts, K, & Porter, K. (2003) How do you size a nasopharyngeal airway. *Resuscitation* **56,** 19–23.

Ryan, A, Larsen, P, Galletly, D. (2003) Comparison of heart rate variability in supine, and left and right lateral positions. *Anaesthesia* **58,** 432–436.

Salem, M, Sellick, B, Elam, J. (1974) The historical background of cricoid pressure in anesthesia and resuscitation. *Anesthes Analg* **53,** 230–232.

Sellick, B. (1961) Cricoid pressure to control regurgitation of stomach contents during induction of anaesthesia. *Lancet* **2,** 404–406.

Stoneham, M. (1993) The nasopharyngeal airway. Assessment and position by fibreoptic laryngoscopy. *Anaesthesia* **48,** 575–580.

Turner, S, Turner, I, Chapman, D *et al.* (1997) A comparative study of the 1992 and 1997 recovery positions for use in the UK. *Resuscitation* **39,** 153–160.

Vanner, R. (1993) Mechanisms of regurgitation and its prevention with cricoid pressure. *Int J Obst Anesthesia* **2,** 207–215.

Vanner, R. (2001) Techniques of cricoid pressure. *Anaesthesia & Intensive Care Medicine* **2,** 362–362.

Vanner, R, & Asai, T. (1999) Safe use of cricoid pressure. *Anaesthesia* **54,** 1–3.

Vanner, R, & Jevon, P. (2002) *Principles of cricoid pressure* (poster).

Vanner, R, & Pryle, B. (1992) Regurgitation and oesophageal rupture with cricoid pressure: a cadaver study. *Anaesthesia* **47,** 732–735.

APPENDIX 1 TRACHEAL INTUBATION

Tracheal intubation is the optimum method of providing and maintaining a clear airway (Nolan *et al.*, 2005). It may be required if basic interventions have been unsuccessful or if there is a risk the airway could become severely compromised. The procedure requires considerable skill and experience and is not without risk (Jevon, 2006). In some patients attempted tracheal intubation may actually lead to life-threatening deterioration, e.g. acute epiglottis pathology, cervical spine injury and head injury (straining could further increase intracranial pressure) (Nolan *et al.*, 2005).

Indications for tracheal intubation include to:

- Secure and maintain a patent airway
- Prevent aspiration of gastric contents
- Facilitate delivery of positive pressure ventilation
- Enable delivery of high concentrations of oxygen.

(Adam & Osborne, 2005)

Tracheal intubation is usually performed by an anaesthetist. However, in order to be an effective assistant, it would be helpful if nurses are familiar with the procedure. The procedure for tracheal intubation will now be described:

- Ensure that all the necessary emergency equipment is immediately available and in working order. The anaesthetist will also usually request drugs to induce anaesthesia, e.g. midazolam (sedative), propofol (muscle relaxant).
- Ensure that the bed is away from the back wall and remove the backrest.
- Attach the patient to a pulse oximeter and an ECG monitor.
- Adopt a position at the top of the bed facing the patient with the feet in the walk/stand position (Resuscitation Council (UK), 2001).
- Pre-oxygenate the patient with at least 85% oxygen for a minimum of 15s.
- Ensure the patient is in the supine position with the neck slightly flexed and the head extended; a pillow under the head and shoulders can help to maintain this position (Jevon, 2006).
- Activate the light in the laryngoscope (if it is the screw-in bulb type, ensure that the bulb is screwed firmly in first).
- Holding the laryngoscope in the left hand, gently insert it into the right side of the patient's mouth, taking care that the lower lip is not caught between the teeth and the blade (Figure 2.11) (Jevon, 2006).
- Advance the laryngoscope blade into the mouth, sweeping the tongue to the left in the process, and position the tip in the

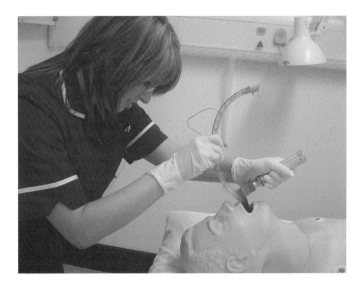

Fig 2.11 Tracheal intubation: holding the laryngoscope in the left hand, gently insert it into the right side of the patient's mouth, taking care that the lower lip is not caught between the teeth and the blade

vallecula (this is the area between the back of the tongue and the base of the epiglottis).

- Lift the laryngoscope upwards along the line of its handle. This will help to lift the epiglottis out of the line of view, revealing the vocal cords. Suction if necessary.
- Insert a lubricated tracheal tube from the right-hand side of the patient's mouth through the vocal cords. The cuff should be positioned just below the vocal cords.
- Inflate the cuff with sufficient air (usually 7–10 ml) to stop the audible leak associated with ventilation.
- Connect to a ventilatory device, e.g. self-inflating bag, ventilator, via a catheter mount.
- Ventilate with high-flow oxygen.
- Confirm that the tracheal tube is correctly placed (see below). If air entry is detected only in the right side of the chest, the

tube may have been inserted too far and is in the right bron-chus: deflate the cuff, withdraw the tube 1–2 cm, re-inflate cuff and reassess (Resuscitation Council UK, 2000).

- Secure the tracheal tube and continue ventilation.
- Regularly reassess the position of the tracheal tube and the effectiveness of ventilation.
- Adopt a comfortable position and avoid prolonged static pos-tures if manually ventilating the patient (Resuscitation Council UK, 2001).
- Tracheal intubation should not exceed 30 s (Nolan *et al.*, 2005).

If undertaking tracheal intubation in a patient who is on the floor:

- Kneel behind the head of the patient, ensuring the knees are a shoulder-width apart
- Bend forwards from the hips over the patient's head
- Resting the elbows on the floor may provide a more stable position.

(Resuscitation Council UK, 2001)

Confirmation of correct tracheal tube placement

Clinical signs of correct tracheal tube placement (e.g. tube con-densation, chest rise, breath sounds on chest auscultation and inability to hear gas sounds entering the stomach) are not 100% reliable (Nolan *et al.*, 2005). As well as performing the standard checks, the use of capnography or an oesophageal detector device will help to minimize the risk of undetected oesophageal intubation:

- *Capnography*: measures the carbon dioxide levels in the patient's exhaled air; <2% indicates oesophageal intubation.
- *Oesophageal detector device*: attach a 50-ml syringe to the tracheal tube and quickly draw back the plunger; easy aspiration indi-cates the tube is in the trachea (difficult aspiration indicates it is in the oesophagus).

(Gwinnutt, 2006)

DOPE

The main causes of ineffective ventilation can be described by the acronym DOPE:

- **D**isplaced tube. Either into pharynx/oesophagus, right/left main bronchus.
- **O**bstructed tube. Vomit, blood, secretions and kinked tube.
- **P**neumothorax.
- **E**quipment failure.

(Jevon, 2006)

APPENDIX 2 RELIEVING A FOREIGN BODY AIRWAY OBSTRUCTION

Foreign body airway obstruction (FBAO) (choking) is a life-threatening emergency. As most FBAO events are associated with eating, they are commonly witnessed, thus providing an opportunity for early intervention while the patient is still conscious (Handley *et al.*, 2005).

Recognition of FBAO

Complete FBAO is often characterized by a sudden inability to talk, maximal respiratory effort, development of cyanosis and clutching of the neck. In partial airway obstruction, the patient will be distressed, may cough and may have a wheeze. In complete airway obstruction, the casualty will be unable to speak, breathe or cough and will eventually collapse and go unconscious. Always ask the patient 'are you choking?' (Handley *et al.*, 2005). If he responds 'yes' by nodding his head without speaking, this indicates severe airway obstruction requiring urgent treatment (American Heart Association, 2005).

FBAO algorithm

If the patient is choking, but able to breathe, encourage him to cough.

If the patient is choking, but is unable to breathe or is displaying signs of becoming weak or stops breathing or coughing, immediate intervention is required.

Procedure

- Stand at side, slightly behind the patient.
- Support his chest with one hand and lean him well forward. This will help ensure that if the foreign body is dislodged, it will drop out of the mouth instead of slipping further down the airway.
- Deliver up to five back blows between the scapulae using the heel of the hand. After each back blow, check to see if it has been successful at relieving the obstruction.
- If the back blows fail, proceed to abdominal thrusts.
- Stand behind the patient, placing both arms around his upper abdomen.
- Lean the patient forward.
- Place a clenched fist between the patient's umbilicus and xiphisternum and clasp it with the other hand.
- Deliver up to five sharp thrusts to the abdomen, inwards and upwards.
- If the obstruction remains, continue alternating five back blows with five chest abdominal thrusts.

If the patient loses consciousness:

- Carefully support him to the ground
- Immediately alert the emergency services
- Start cardiopulmonary resuscitation: 30 chest compressions first (even if there is a pulse) – chest compressions may relieve the obstruction

(Source: Handley *et al.*, 2005)

APPENDIX 3 APPLICATION OF CRICOID PRESSURE

Cricoid pressure (Sellick's manoeurvre) is the application of backward pressure on the cricoid cartilage (Sellick, 1961), providing a physical barrier to regurgitation of gastric contents (Gwinnutt, 2006). It can sometimes be helpful during a difficult tracheal intubation (Jevon, 2006).

The cricoid cartilage, situated below the thyroid cartilage, is the only complete ring of cartilage in the respiratory system (Koziol *et al.*, 2000). The other tracheal cartilages are c-shaped (i.e. incomplete rings of cartilage), which could collapse if pressure is applied (Feinstein & Owens, 1992). When correctly applied, cricoid pressure compresses the proximal oesophageal lumen between the cricoid cartilage and the cervical vertebrae (Vanner, 1993) occluding the lumen of the oesophagus, which helps to prevent regurgitation and aspiration of gastric contents.

The application of cricoid pressure can help prevent the passive regurgitation and aspiration of gastric contents. Indications include:

- Emergency induction of general anaesthesia (i.e. patient has not been fasted)
- Induction of anaesthesia for caesarean section
- Sometimes during attempted tracheal intubation.

(Jevon, 2006)

There is an increased risk of regurgitation in pregnancy, in obese patients and in patients with a 'full stomach', even those that have been fasted prior to surgery if there is delayed gastric emptying, e.g. bowel obstruction, opiate administration and trauma (Koziol *et al.*, 2000).

30 N (3 kg) of pressure needs to be applied to the cricoid cartilage to occlude the oesophagus (Vanner & Pryle, 1992) (less is applied prior to induction). Practically, this roughly equates to sufficient pressure on the bridge of the nose to cause pain (Mehrotra and Paust, 1979) or sufficient pressure on the cricoid to prevent swallowing (Gutsche, 1993).

- Position a pillow underneath the patient's head and shoulders.
- Locate the cricoid cartilage – this is the first complete ring of cartilage below the thyroid cartilage (Adam's apple).
- Place the index finger and thumb of the dominant hand on either side of the cricoid cartilage.

- Apply cricoid pressure as advised by the anaesthetist. Following pre-oxygenation, but prior to intravenous induction, apply a force of 10N (1 kg) and once the patient loses consciousness apply a force of 30N (3 kg).
- If cervical spine injury is suspected, apply counter pressure to the back of the neck (to reduce movement of the cervical spine).
- Release cricoid pressure once a cuffed tracheal tube protects the airway, if the patient actively vomits or on the anaesthetist's request (Jevon, 2006).
- If lung inflation is difficult, reduce the pressure being applied or release the pressure completely (Nolan *et al.*, 2005).

(Source: Jevon, 2006)

Complications of cricoid pressure include:

- Retching and death from aspiration and ruptured oesophagus if excess force applied in a patient who is awake
- Difficult tracheal intubation
- Difficult ventilation
- Aggravation of an existing cervical spine injury.

(Heath *et al.*, 1996)

3 | Treating a Patient with Compromised Breathing

INTRODUCTION

Breathing can be compromised by a lung disorder, e.g. asthma, or by any condition that leads to a decrease in respiratory drive, e.g. drugs, or a decrease in respiratory effort, e.g. Guillan–Barré syndrome (Resuscitation Council UK, 2006). If the patient's breathing is compromised, hypoxia and hypoxaemia can develop. Some vital organs, e.g. brain and kidneys, are more susceptible to, and rapidly damaged by, sustained hypoxia and hypoxaemia (Leech, 2004). If untreated, compromised breathing could lead to cardiopulmonary arrest. Early detection and correction of tissue hypoxia is paramount if progressive organ dysfunction and death are to be avoided (Leech & Treacher, 2002).

It is therefore essential to be able to recognize that the patient's breathing is compromised. A comprehensive assessment of breathing has been described in Chapter 1. The patient will usually present with signs of respiratory distress, e.g. tachypnoea, though sometimes may present with bradypnoea, which could be a sign of imminent cardiopulmonary arrest. The priorities of treatment are to administer high concentrations of oxygen and to identify and effectively treat the underlying cause; sometimes assisted ventilation will be required.

The aim of this chapter is to help in understanding the treatment of a patient with compromised breathing.

LEARNING OBJECTIVES

At the end of this chapter the reader will be able to:

❏ List the causes of compromised breathing
❏ Discuss the classification of cyanosis

❏ Describe the signs and clinical features of breathlessness
❏ Outline the principles of oxygen therapy.

CAUSES OF COMPROMISED BREATHING

Causes of compromised breathing include:

- Lung disease, e.g. asthma, pneumonia, acute exacerbation of chronic obstructive pulmonary disease (COPD).
- Lung function disorders, e.g. tension pneumothorax, pulmonary embolism, pulmonary oedema.
- Reduced respiratory drive caused by central nervous system (CNS) depression. Causes include drugs, e.g. opiates, and a cerebral insult.
- Reduced respiratory effort caused by muscle weakness or nerve damage, e.g. myasthenia gravis, multiple sclerosis and Guillan–Barré syndrome.

(Source: Resuscitation Council UK, 2006)

CLASSIFICATION OF CYANOSIS

Cyanosis can be defined as a blue discoloration of the skin and mucous membranes resulting from an inadequate amount of oxygen in the blood (McFerran & Martin, 2003). If the patient is peripherally blue, but centrally pink, this is termed peripheral cyanosis. If the patient is centrally blue, this is termed central cyanosis.

Peripheral cyanosis

Peripheral cyanosis (cold, blue fingers) is caused by peripheral circulatory failure resulting in excessive oxygen extraction from the capillaries (Ford *et al.*, 2005). Causes of peripheral circulatory failure include shock, hypovolaemia, cold ambient temperature and arterial or venous obstruction.

Central cyanosis

Central cyanosis (blue tongue, lips and fingers with warm hands) is caused by a central failure of oxygen transfer across the lung alveolar-capillary membranes (Ford *et al.*, 2005). It will be evident if the PO_2 is < 8 kPa (55 mg/Hg), an oxygen saturation of 85% (Gwinnutt, 2006). As cyanosis is usually detectable in polycythaemic patients, but not in anaemic patients (Smith, 2003), it is a poor indicator of hypoxia (Leach, 2004).

Causes of central cyanosis

Central cyanosis can be associated with airway obstruction, respiratory compromise and heart failure (McFerran & Martin, 2003). Causes of central cyanosis include:

- *Hypoventilation*: causes include CNS disorders, e.g. head injury; CNS depressant drugs, e.g. opiates; airway obstruction; and neuromuscular disorders, e.g. Guillan–Barré syndrome
- *Ventilation–perfusion mismatch*: causes include pulmonary oedema, severe acute asthma and pulmonary embolism
- *Impaired transfer of gases*: causes include pulmonary fibrosis and pulmonary oedema
- *Right-to-left intracardiac shunt*: causes include congenital and postmyocardial infarction abnormalities.

(Source: Smith, 2003)

SIGNS AND CLINICAL FEATURES OF COMPROMISED BREATHING

The signs and clinical features of compromised breathing include:

- Tachypnoea
- Tachycardia and a bounding pulse
- Cyanosis or pallor
- Use of accessory muscles of respiration
- Altered consciousness level, e.g. agitation, confusion and restlessness
- Low oxygen saturation levels.

(Sources: Jevon & Ewens, 2002 and
Shelly & Nightingale, 1999)

The assessment of respiratory function is discussed in detail in Chapter 1.

The most common causes of compromised breathing that herald avoidable cardiopulmonary arrest are:

- Acute asthma
- Pulmonary oedema
- Exacerbation of COPD
- Pulmonary embolism
- Bronchopneumonia
- Shock.

(Hodgetts *et al.*, 2004)

An overview of the emergency treatment of these potentially life-threatening conditions is included on page 67.

PRINCIPLES OF OXYGEN THERAPY

Oxygen therapy can be life saving when safely and correctly administered (Bateman & Leach, 1998). Oxygen is a drug which should be prescribed by an appropriately trained practitioner (Jamieson *et al.*, 2002), although in the emergency situation, it should be administered without delay (Higgins, 2005).

All critically ill patients should receive oxygen (Resuscitation Council UK, 2006). Oxygen is administered to treat hypoxaemia and should initially be of a high concentration, which can then be adjusted according to the results of pulse oximetry and arterial blood gas analysis (Shelly & Nightingale, 1999). The administration of oxygen does not replace the definitive treatment of the underlying condition (Oh, 2004).

Aim of oxygen therapy

The aim of oxygen therapy is to supplement inspired oxygen concentration to prevent tissue hypoxia and the resultant cellular dysfunction (Higgins, 2005). The treatment for hypoxaemia is the administration of high concentrations of oxygen, ideally to achieve a normal PaO_2 (12–14 kPa) or normal peripheral oxygen saturation (95%) (Gwinnutt, 2006). In patients with COPD, a PaO_2

of 8 kPa or peripheral oxygen saturation of 90–92% is acceptable (see below) (Resuscitation Council UK, 2006).

Cellular oxygen delivery is dependent upon inspired oxygen, haemoglobin levels and its ability to saturate with oxygen, and cardiac output (Higgins, 2005). Although the administration of supplementary oxygen can be life saving in some situations, it cannot correct inadequate oxygen delivery caused by a low cardiac output or impaired ventilation (Leach & Treacher, 2002). Oxygen delivery therefore needs to be supported (e.g. patent airway, adequate breathing and adequate circulation) in order to help avoid tissue hypoxia, end-organ damage and high mortality rates (Levy, 2005).

Clinical indications for oxygen therapy

Clinical indications for oxygen therapy include:

- Breathless patient
- Low oxygen saturation
- Cardiopulmonary arrest
- Respiratory failure (types 1 and 2) (Box 3.1)
- Acute coronary syndrome
- Heart failure
- Increased metabolic demands, e.g. burns, multiple injuries and sepsis
- Postoperative period
- Carbon monoxide poisoning.

(Jevon & Ewens, 2002 and Oh, 2004)

Box 3.1 Types of respiratory failure

Type 1 respiratory failure: hypoxaemia without CO_2 retention, e.g. asthma, pulmonary oedema, pulmonary embolism and pneumonia

Type 2 respiratory failure: hypoxaemia with CO_2 retention, e.g. chronic obstructive airways disease, chest trauma, postoperative hypoxaemia, drug-induced unconsciousness

(Oh, 2004)

Oxygen therapy in patients with COPD

Excessive oxygen administration in patients with severe COPD (classically described as 'blue bloaters') can predispose to worsening respiratory failure (Ting, 2004 and Gwinnutt, 2006). The concern is that the administration of high concentrations of oxygen will remove the respiratory drive, resulting in hypoventilation with rising hypercapnia, leading to unconsciousness and respiratory arrest (Gwinnutt, 2006).

However, although high concentrations of oxygen could depress breathing in patients with COPD, these patients could sustain end-organ damage or cardiopulmonary arrest should their blood oxygen levels be allowed to fall (Resuscitation Council UK, 2006). Patients do not die of hypercapnia, they die of hypoxia: patients will die because high concentrations of oxygen have been withheld due to an unwarranted concern about hypoxic respiratory drive (Gwinnutt, 2006). The correction of hypoxia overrides strategies to avert oxygen-related hypercapnia (Ting, 2004).

In patients with COPD, the aim of oxygen therapy is to achieve a PaO_2 of 8 kPa or peripheral oxygen saturation of 90–92% (Resuscitation Council UK, 2006).

Monitoring oxygen therapy

Oxygen therapy can be monitored by arterial blood gas analysis and by pulse oximetry (Figure 3.1): arterial blood gas analysis provides accurate information on the pH, PaO_2 and $PaCO_2$ (i.e. effectiveness of ventilation), while pulse oximetry provides continuous monitoring of the state of oxygenation (Jevon & Ewens, 2002).

If the patient fails to improve with oxygen therapy, senior help should be sought: the patient may require assistance with his breathing, e.g. continuous positive airway pressure (CPAP), non-invasive or invasive positive pressure ventilation (Gwinnutt, 2006).

Dangers of oxygen therapy

Dangers of oxygen therapy include:

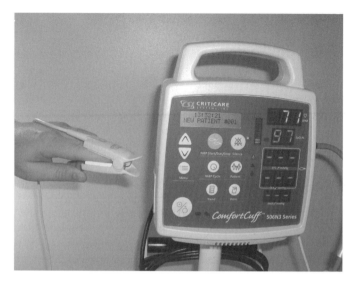

Fig 3.1 Pulse oximetry

- *Hypercapnia due to hypoventilation*: 10% of breathless patients, mainly COPD, have type 2 respiratory failure and 40–50% of patients with COPD are at risk of type 2 respiratory failure (see Box 3.1)
- *Fire*: ensure that no part of the cylinder or equipment is either lubricated or contaminated with oil or grease and that there is no smoking/naked flames in the vicinity (BOC Medical, 2001)
- *Pulmonary oxygen toxicity*: high concentrations of oxygen (>60%) for prolonged periods (24–48 h) can lead to damage of the alveolar membranes causing acute respiratory distress syndrome (Leach, 2004).

Local guidelines on oxygen therapy

The availability of local guidelines on the use of oxygen therapy improves the effectiveness of oxygen administration, improves the effective use of pulse oximetry and increases the nurse's awareness of the importance of close monitoring of patients with respiratory disease (Kar & Campbell, 2006).

OXYGEN DELIVERY SYSTEMS

Non-rebreathing mask

A non-rebreathing mask with an oxygen reservoir bag (Figure 3.2) can be used to deliver high concentrations of oxygen to a patient who is spontaneously breathing. Its use is recommended in critically ill patients (Resuscitation Council UK, 2006).

A one-way valve diverts the oxygen flow into the reservoir bag during expiration; then during inspiration the contents of the reservoir bag, together with the high-flow oxygen, results in minimal entrainment of air and an inspired oxygen concentration of approximately 85% (Gwinnutt, 2006). The valve also prevents the patient's exhaled gases from entering the reservoir bag.

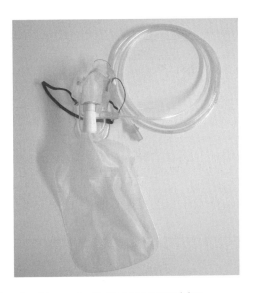

Fig 3.2 Non-rebreathing mask with an oxygen reservoir bag

The use of the oxygen reservoir bag helps to increase the inspired oxygen concentration by preventing oxygen loss during inspiration (Leech, 2004).

It is important to ensure that a sufficient oxygen flow rate is used to ensure that the oxygen reservoir bag does not collapse during inspiration (Resuscitation Council UK, 2006). Some non-rebreathing masks have elasticated earloop bands, which are ideal for trauma patents, because the head can remain still while the mask is applied.

The following procedure is recommended when using a non-rebreathing mask:

- Attach the tubing to the oxygen source and set the oxygen flow rate to 15l/min (Figure 3.3a) (Smith, 2003)
- Occlude the valve between the mask and the oxygen reservoir bag (Figure 3.3b) and check that the bag fills up with oxygen
- Squeeze the oxygen reservoir bag (Figure 3.3c) to check the patency of the valve between the mask and the reservoir bag: if the reservoir bag does not empty, discard it and choose another (Smith, 2003)

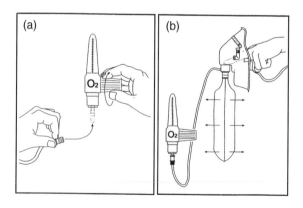

Fig 3.3a Attach the tubing to the oxygen source and set the oxygen flow rate to 15 l/min

Fig 3.3b Occlude the valve between the mask and the oxygen reservoir bag to check that the bag fills up with oxygen (Diagrams reproduced courtesy of Intersurgical)

- Again occlude the valve between the mask and the oxygen reservoir bag (Figure 3.3a), allowing the latter to fill up
- Place the mask with a filled oxygen reservoir bag on the patient's face, ensuring a tight fit (Figure 3.4d) (Smith, 2003).

Some masks have a respiratory rate indicator (Figure 3.3e). This indicator can be affected by:

- The patient's respiratory rate
- The orientation of the indicator
- The oxygen flow rate
- The fit of the mask to the patient's face
- The presence of moisture in the indicator tube – this can actually stop the indicator from working.

(Intersurgical, 2003)

The respiratory rate indicator should only be used as a guide and should not replace close monitoring of the patient's breathing.

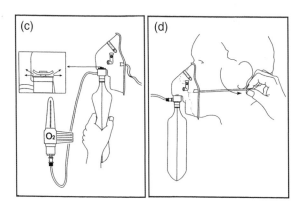

Fig 3.3c Squeeze the oxygen reservoir bag to check the patency of the valve between the mask and the reservoir bag

Fig 3.3d Place the mask with a filled oxygen reservoir bag on the patient's face, ensuring a tight fit (Diagrams reproduced courtesy of Intersurgical)

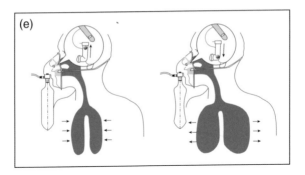

Fig 3.3e Some masks have a respiratory rate indicator (Diagram reproduced courtesy of Intersurgical)

Fixed performance mask

A fixed performance mask is used when it is important to deliver a precise concentration of oxygen, which is unaffected by the patient's ventilatory pattern (Gwinnutt, 2006). These masks, sometimes referred to as high airflow oxygen enrichment (HAFOE) masks or venturi masks, incorporate a venturi barrel, providing a higher gas flow than the patient's peak inspiratory flow rate. Exhalation holes on the mask ensure that expired gas is flushed out, resulting in minimal rebreathing and little increase in dead space (Flexicare, 2006).

A fixed performance mask may deliver either a fixed percentage of oxygen, e.g. 40%, or it may have interchangeable, usually colour-coded, venturi heads (Figure 3.4), allowing it to deliver varying percentages of oxygen dependent upon the particular venturi head used. The percentage of oxygen delivered is dependent upon the flow of oxygen via the inlet and the size of the holes through which air is entrained (Higgins, 2005).

Variable performance devices

Variable performance devices, e.g. simple face mask, nasal cannula, are usually sufficient for patients who just require some supplementary oxygen, e.g. post anaesthesia. The precise amount of oxygen delivered is not known because it will be dependent

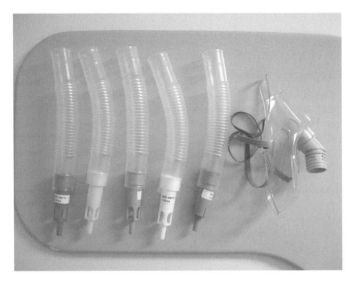

Fig 3.4 Colour-coded venturi heads allowing the delivery of varying percentages of oxygen

upon the patient's respiratory pattern and the oxygen flow rate selected (Gwinnutt, 2006). These devices are not usually used in critically ill patients.

Nasal cannulae (sometimes referred to as nasal prongs or specs) can be helpful if the patient is unable to tolerate a face-mask. They consist of two prongs that are gently inserted inside the patient's anterior nares. A cannula is more comfortable and more easily tolerated than a mask and it delivers a constant flow of oxygen.

Even if the patient is breathing through his mouth, oxygen delivered via a nasal cannula is still inhaled (Leech, 2004). Lower oxygen flow rates are used, usually 2–4 l/min, resulting in an inspired oxygen concentration of approximately 25–40% (Gwinnutt, 2006). Higher oxygen flow rates are sometimes used. However, this can quickly lead to discomfort and dryness of the nasal mucosa (Pierce, 1995) and nasal cannulae cannot be connected satisfactorily to an external humidification device (Dougherty & Lister, 2005).

Oxygen humidification

During normal breathing, inspired air is humidified, heated and filtered (Pilkington, 2004). However, the efficacy of this process can be significantly reduced by a number of factors, including prolonged mouth breathing, respiratory tract infection, oxygen therapy, dehydration and room temperature (Fowler, 2000). If the patient has a tracheal tube *in situ* or has a tracheostomy, injury to the respiratory tract can be caused after only 3 h (Oh, 2004). Oxygen humidification should therefore be considered in critically ill patients on prolonged oxygen therapy.

There are several methods available to provide humidification of oxygen, depending upon the circumstances:

- *Cold water humidifier*: oxygen is passed through a room temperature water reservoir (Branson, 2003)
- *Hot water humidifier*: oxygen is passed through a heated water humidifier or an adjustable aerosol heater (Pilkington, 2004)
- *Heat moisture exchangers (HME)*: rely on heat and moisture in the patient's expired air being retained in paper or foam, which then returns to the patient during inspiration (Pilkington, 2004)
- *Nebulization*: produces an aerosol of water droplets to humidify the inspired gases (Branson, 2003).

(Source: Pilkington, 2004)

Potential problems of humidification include:

- Excess water can result in fluid overload and increased airway resistance
- Excess heat can lead to a rise in the patient's core temperature and airway burns
- Blockage of the tubing
- Infection arising in the water reservoir.

(Pilkington, 2004)

NON-INVASIVE AND INVASIVE VENTILATION

Non-invasive ventilation

Non-invasive ventilation, which refers to ventilatory support without tracheal intubation, can be used as a first step in patients who need some ventilatory support, but are not severely hypoxaemic (Shelly & Nightingale, 1999). It reduces the work of breathing, improves cardiac function, increases tissue oxygen delivery and may prevent the need for tracheal intubation (Leech, 2004).

Non-invasive ventilation is most successful in a patient who is alert, co-operative, self-inflating, haemodynamically stable and who can clear and maintain his own airway (Leach, 2004). In patients with acute COPD, non-invasive ventilation results in reduced morbidity and mortality if it is used first before considering tracheal intubation (Gwinnutt, 2006).

Indications for non-invasive ventilation include:

- Acute COPD
- Respiratory failure when tracheal intubation is considered inappropriate, e.g. end-stage respiratory disease.

(Leach, 2004)

CPAP

CPAP (Figure 3.5) is when a breathing system is connected to a tightly fitted facemask and a continuous positive pressure (usually 5–10 cm H_2O) is maintained during both inspiration and expiration (Leach, 2004). The CPAP mask may only cover the nose: this is termed nasal CPAP (Gwinnutt, 2006). CPAP improves oxygenation by:

- Increasing functional residual capacity
- Re-expanding areas of the lungs that have collapsed
- Reducing the incidence of lung collapse during expiration.

(Gwinnutt, 2006)

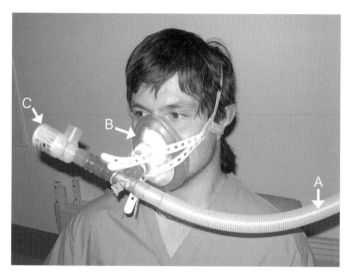

Fig 3.5 Continuous positive airways pressure (CPAP)

BIPAP

Bilevel positive airways pressure (BIPAP) is when two levels of CPAP are delivered. The higher pressure facilitates alveolar ventilation and CO_2 clearance, while the lower pressure helps prevent alveolar collapse (Leach, 2004).

Invasive ventilation

Invasive ventilation is when the patient is anaesthetized, intubated and sedated so that he can tolerate the tracheal tube; full mechanical ventilation will be required and the patient will need to be managed on an ICU (Gwinnutt, 2005).

Clinical findings confirming the imminent requirement for invasive ventilation include:

- Hypoxaemia ($PaO_2 < 8\,kPa$ or $SaO_2 < 90\%$) despite the delivery of maximum oxygen therapy

- Hypercapnoea with deterioration in the level of consciousness
- Falling in vital capacity in patients with neuromuscular disorders.

(Shelley & Nightingale, 1999)

If the patient has acute respiratory failure, which has not been caused by COPD, ICU admission and invasive ventilation will usually be required, particularly when multiple organ system failure is present (Gwinnutt, 2006).

VENTILATION WITH A POCKET MASK AND SELF-INFLATING BAG DEVICE

If the patient's breathing is inadequate or absent, call for expert help (usually dial 2222 for the cardiac arrest team), and begin ventilation (Resuscitation Council UK, 2006). Effective ventilation and oxygenation will help to preserve cerebral function. Every nurse must be competent at providing effective ventilations using locally available resources. In hospital, at the very least, a pocket mask should always be immediately available (Soar & Spearpoint, 2005). The self-inflating bag device is commonly used. Ventilation with a pocket mask and a self-inflating bag device will now be described.

Ventilation with a pocket mask

The pocket mask (Figure 3.6), an excellent first response device, is transparent, thus facilitating prompt detection of vomit or blood in the patient's airway. A one-way valve directs the patient's expired air away from the nurse (Jevon, 2006).

The pocket mask usually has an oxygen connector for the attachment of supplementary oxygen (10l/min) (Resuscitation Council UK, 2006), enabling an inspired oxygen concentration of approximately 50% to be achieved (Jevon, 2006). If there is no oxygen connector, supplementary oxygen can still be added by placing the oxygen tubing underneath one side of the mask and pressing down to achieve a seal (Nolan *et al.*, 2005).

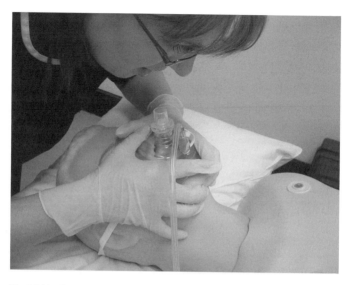

Fig 3.6 Ventilation using a pocket mask

A suggested procedure for pocket mask ventilation:

- Don gloves (if available).
- Kneel behind the patient's head, ensuring the knees are a shoulder-width apart (if alone kneel at the side of the patient level with his nose and mouth) (Resuscitation Council UK, 2001).
- Rest back to sit on the knees and adopt a low kneeling position (Resuscitation Council UK, 2001).
- Bend forwards from the hips, leaning down towards the patient's face and resting the elbows on your legs to support your weight (Resuscitation Council UK, 2001).
- If available, attach oxygen to the oxygen connector on the mask at a rate of 10l/min (Resuscitation Council UK, 2006). If there is no oxygen connector, place the oxygen tubing underneath one side of the mask and press down to achieve a seal (Nolan *et al.*, 2005).

- Apply the mask to the patient's face; press down with the thumbs and lift the chin into the mask by applying pressure behind the angles of the jaw.
- Take a breath in and ventilate the patient with sufficient air to cause visible chest rise. Each ventilation should last 1 s.
- If the patient is on a bed or trolley, stand at the side facing the patient, level with his nose and mouth, and bend forwards from the hips to minimize flexion of the spine; the nurse's weight can also be supported by resting the elbows on the bed and leaning the legs against the side of the bed frame (Figure 3.6) (Resuscitation Council UK, 2001).
- Always adopt a comfortable position for ventilation and avoid static postures (Resuscitation Council UK, 2001).

(Source: Jevon, 2006)

Ventilation with a self-inflating bag device

The self-inflating bag device allows the delivery of higher concentrations of oxygen. If an oxygen reservoir bag is attached, with an oxygen flow rate of 10 l/min, an inspired oxygen concentration of approximately 85% can be achieved (Nolan *et al.*, 2005).

However, its use by a single person requires considerable skill (Jevon, 2006). When used with a face-mask, it can be difficult to achieve a seal with the mask, maintain an open airway and squeeze the bag (Alexander *et al.*, 1993). A two-person technique is therefore recommended, one person to open the airway and ensure a good seal with the mask, while the other squeezes the bag (Figure 3.7) (Nolan *et al.*, 2005).

A suggested procedure for ventilation with a self-inflating bag device is:

- Ensure the patient is supine.
- Move the bed away from the wall and remove the backrest, if applicable.
- Adopt a position at the top of the bed facing the patient, with the feet in a walk/stand position (Resuscitation Council UK, 2001).

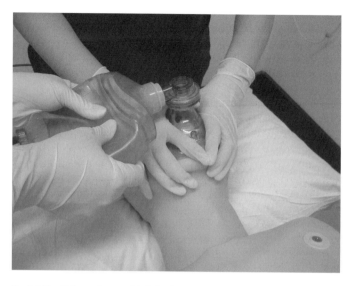

Fig 3.7 Ventilation using a self-inflating bag device

- Select an appropriately sized mask. It should comfortably cover the mouth and nose (not the eyes) and should not override the chin.
- Attach oxygen reservoir bag and connect oxygen at a flow rate of 10 l/min (Nolan *et al.*, 2005).
- First nurse: tilt the head back, apply the mask to the face and press down on it using the thumbs. Lift the chin into the mask by applying pressure behind the angles of the jaw. The patient's airway should now be open and an adequate face/mask seal achieved. A pillow under the head and shoulders can help to maintain this position.
- Second nurse (positioned to the side of the bed): squeeze the bag (not the oxygen reservoir bag) sufficiently to cause visible chest rise; each ventilation should be delivered over 1 s.
- Observe for chest movement. If the chest does not rise, recheck the patency of the airway; slight readjustment may be all that is required (Jevon, 2006).

- Adopt a comfortable position for ventilation and avoid static postures. Supporting your weight by resting your elbows on the bed may help (Resuscitation Council UK, 2001).

(Source: Jevon, 2006)

Minimising gastric inflation

Excessive tidal volumes or inspiratory flows can generate excessive airway pressures, which can lead to gastric inflation and the subsequent risk of regurgitation and aspiration of gastric contents (Nolan *et al.*, 2005). It is therefore recommended to deliver each ventilation over 1 s, with sufficient volume to achieve chest rise, but avoiding rapid and forceful ventilations (Handley *et al.*, 2005).

Ineffective ventilations

If ventilations fail to achieve chest rise:

- Ensure adequate head tilt and chin lift
- Recheck the patient's mouth and remove any obstruction
- Ensure there is a good seal between the mask and the patient's face.

(Jevon, 2006)

TREATMENT OF A BREATHLESS PATIENT

The treatment of a breathless patient includes:

- Call for expert help.
- Position the patient in an upright position to maximize chest expansion
- Request pulse oximetry and monitor oxygen saturation levels.
- Initially administer high concentrations of oxygen. This should ideally be prescribed. Use a non-rebreathe mask with an oxygen reservoir bag connected to an oxygen flow rate of 15 l/min (Smith, 2003).
- Reduce oxygen consumption, e.g. cooling, analgesia, sedation, reassurance to help reduce anxiety and prevention of shivering (Leech, 2004)

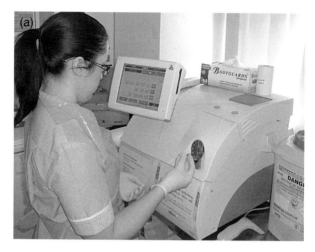

PH	7.35–7.45
PaCO₂	4.7–6.0 kPa
PaO₂	12.5–13.0 kPa
HCO₃	22–26 mmols
BE	+2 mmols– ⁻2 mmols

Fig 3.8a Arterial blood gas analysis
Fig 3.8b Normal blood gas results (Source: Resuscitation Council UK, 2006)

- Monitor the effect of oxygen therapy and any other interventions.
- If available, use capnography.
- Perform arterial blood gas analysis (Figure 3.8a) to assess the effectiveness of ventilation. Normal blood gas results are depicted in Figure 3.8b.
- Check the patient's drug prescription chart – have any medications been administered which may compromise breathing? e.g. an opiate can lead to respiratory depression.

- Identify and treat the underlying cause of the breathlessness. Oxygen therapy alone does not treat the cause of hypoxaemia and respiratory failure: the next step is to identify and effectively treat the cause (Gwinnutt, 2006) (Box 3.2).
- If ventilation is inadequate, begin assisted ventilation using a ventilatory device, e.g. pocket mask, self-inflating bag.

Box 3.2 Specific treatment of tachypnoea

Acute asthma: salbutamol 5 mg via nebulizer (repeated as necessary) and hydrocortisone 200 mg i.v.; ipratropium 500 mg via nebulizer, i.v. salbutamol, i.v. magnesium, i.v. aminophyline may also be considered

Pulmonary oedema: if systolic blood pressure > 90 mmHg administer two puffs of glyceryl trinitrate spray sublingual and then start i.v. nitrates, i.v. frusemide, i.v. opiate together with metaclopramide 10 mg i.v. – opiate should be used with extreme caution

Pulmonary embolism (PE): anti-coagulation therapy, if massive PE, i.v. fluids and thrombolytic therapy may be required

Exacerbation of COPD: controlled administration of oxygen guided by arterial blood gas analysis, antibiotics if chest infection present and treat bronchospasm if necessary (see treatment for asthma above)

Bronchopneumonia: antibiotics, e.g. amoxicillin and erythromycin (or clarithromycin)

      (Sources: Hodgetts *et al.*, 2004 and Wyatt *et al.*, 2006)

CONCLUSION

Whatever the cause, compromised breathing can lead to life-threatening hypoxia and hypoxaemia. Early detection and correction of tissue hypoxia is paramount if progressive organ dysfunction and death are to be avoided. Initial priorities include administration of high concentrations of oxygen and identifying and treating the underlying cause.

REFERENCES

Alexander, R, Hodgson, P, Lomax, D, Bullen, C. (1993) A comparison of the laryngeal mask airway and guedel airway, bag and face mask for manual ventilation following formal training. *Anaesthesia* **48,** 231–234.

BOC Medical (2001) *Gas Safe.* BOC Medical, Manchester.

Branson, R. (2003) *Humidification Handbook.* Hudson RCI, Sweden.

Flexicare (2006) Oxygen therapy www.flexicare.com (accessed 8 September 2006).

Fowler, S. (2000) Know how: a guide to humidification. *Nursing Times* **96,** 10–11 (High Dependency suppl.).

Gwinnutt, C. (2006) *Clinical Anaesthesia,* 2nd edn. Blackwell Publishing, Oxford.

Handley, A, Kester, R, Monsieurs, K *et al.* (2005) European Resuscitation Council Guidelines for Resuscitation 2005: Section 2. Adult basic life support and use of automated external defibrillators. *Resuscitation* **67S1,** S7–S23.

Higgins, D. (2005) Oxygen therapy. *Nursing Times* **101,** 30–31.

Hodgetts, T, Ineson, N, Shaikh, L *et al.* (2004) *In-Hospital Cardiac Arrest*: *Treatment Guidelines* www.metproject.org.uk

Intersurgical (2003) *Product literature for Respi Check Mask.* Intersurgical, Wokingham.

Jamieson, E *et al.* (2002) *Clinical Nursing Procedures.* Churchill Livingstone, Edinburgh.

Kar, F & Campbell, I. (2006) Oxygen therapy in hospitalized patients: the impact of local guidelines. *Journal of Evaluation in Clinical Practice* **12,** 31–36.

Leach, R & Treacher, D. (2002) The pulmonary physician in critical care c 2: Oxygen delivery and consumption in the critically ill. *Thorax* **57,** 170–177.

Levy, M. (2005) Pathophysiology of oxygen delivery in respiratory failure. *Chest* **128** (Suppl. 2), 547S–553S.

Nolan, J, Deakin, C, Soar, J *et al.* (2005) European Resuscitation Council Guidelines for Resuscitation 2005: Section 4. Adult advanced life support. *Resuscitation* **675S,** S39–S86.

Pierce, L. (1995) *Guide to Mechanical Ventilation and Intensive Respiratory Care*. WB Saunders, London.

Pilkington, F. (2004) Humidification for oxygen therapy in non-ventilated patients. *Br J Nursing* **13**, 111–115.

Resuscitation Council UK (2001) *Guidance for Safer Handling during Resuscitation in Hospitals*. Resuscitation Council (UK), London.

Resuscitation Council (UK) (2006) *Advanced life Support*, 5th edn. Resuscitation Council (UK), London.

Shelly, M & Nightingale, P. (1999) Respiratory support. In: Singer, M, Grant, I, eds. *ABC of Intensive Care*. BMJ Books, London.

Soar, J & Spearpoint, K. (2005) In-hospital resuscitation. In: *Resuscitation Guidelines 2005*. Resuscitation Council UK, London.

Ting, J. (2004) Hypercapnia and oxygen therapy in older asthmatic patients. *European Journal of Emergency Medicine* **11**, 355–357.

4 | Treating a Patient with Hypotension

INTRODUCTION

Hypotension is symptomatic of shock (Hodgetts *et al.*, 2004). It is common in the critically ill patient, resulting in poor perfusion of the vital organs, e.g. heart, brain and kidney. It is often caused by hypovolaemia, which will often respond well to appropriate fluid resuscitation. If left untreated, the patient's condition will rapidly deteriorate (Ahern & Philpot, 2002).

In shock, hypotension is a late sign and occurs once the compensatory mechanisms, which have been activated in response to hypoperfusion, are overwhelmed (Graham & Parke, 2005). If there is delay in instituting effective treatment, then shock can become established and organ failure supervenes (Leach & Treacher, 2002). Non-traumatic hypotension measured in the emergency department has an increased risk of in-hospital mortality (Jones *et al.*, 2006).

> Hypotension should be regarded as a medical emergency, requiring rapid treatment and identification of the cause (Smith, 2003).

At the end of this chapter the reader will understand how to treat a patient with hypotension.

LEARNING OBJECTIVES

At the end of this chapter the reader will be able to:

❏ Describe the procedure for recording blood pressure (BP)
❏ Define hypotension

❏ Discuss the physiology of hypotension
❏ List the causes of hypotension
❏ Describe the effects of hypotension
❏ Outline shock
❏ Discuss the treatment of hypotension.

PROCEDURE FOR RECORDING BLOOD PRESSURE

Of all the measurements routinely undertaken in clinical practice, the recording of BP is potentially the most unreliably and incorrectly performed (British Hypertensive Society, 2006a). It is essential that BP recordings are accurate and reliable: good practice can significantly reduce measurement errors and help ensure that the BP recording obtained is accurate and reliable.

Systolic and diastolic blood pressure

- *Systolic BP*: peak blood pressure in the artery following ventricular systole (contraction)
- *Diastolic BP*: level to which the arterial BP falls during ventricular diastole (relaxation)

(Talley & O'Connor, 2001)

Korotkoff's sounds

Five different sound phases known as 'Korotkoff's sounds' (Korotkoff, a Russian surgeon, first described the auscultation method of measuring BP in 1905) can be heard as the BP cuff is slowly released:

- Phase 1: A thud
- Phase 2: A blowing or swishing noise
- Phase 3: A softer thud than in sound 1
- Phase 4: A disappearing blowing noise
- Phase 5: Silence

(Sources: Talley & O'Connor, 2001 and
Dougherty & Lister, 2004)

Practically, the systolic reading is when the Korotkoff sounds are first heard and the diastolic reading is when the sounds disappear (British Hypertensive Society, 2006a).

Which arm

The BP should initially be measured in both arms and the arm with the higher readings should be used for subsequent measurements (Beever *et al.*, 2001, MHRA, 2006 and NICE & British Hypertensive Society, 2006). Although a difference in BP measurements between the arms can be expected in 20% of patients, if this difference is > 20 mmHg for systolic or > 10 mmHg for diastolic on three consecutive readings, further investigation will probably be indicated (MHRA, 2006 and NICE & British Hypertensive Society, 2006).

Procedure for manual measurement of a blood pressure

The traditional manual BP device (Figure 4.1) using auscultation is still a very popular and, when used correctly, reliable method of recording BP. The following procedure for its use is recommended:

- Ideally ensure that the patient has been sitting or lying down for at least 5 min and is comfortably relaxed.
- Check the equipment, ensuring it is in good working order.
- Explain the procedure to the patient and obtain his consent.
- Ask the patient to remove any tight clothing from around his arm.
- Ensure the patient's arm is supported at the level of the heart. If the arm is unsupported, the BP is likely to be erroneously increased due to muscle contraction in the arm (Smith, 2003). If the arm is higher than the level of the heart, this can lead to an underestimation of the diastolic pressure by as much as 10 mmHg (MHRA, 2006).
- Select an appropriately sized cuff: the bladder of the cuff should encircle at least 80% of the arm but no more than 100%.

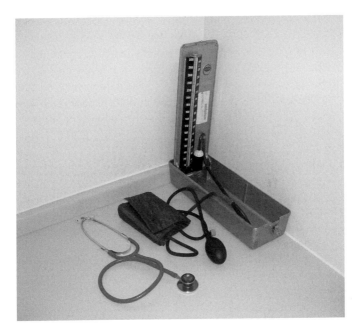

Fig 4.1 Manual blood pressure device

- Place the cuff snugly onto the patient's arm, with the centre of the bladder over the brachial artery – most cuffs have a 'brachial artery indicator', an arrow which should be aligned with the brachial artery.
- Position the manometer near to the patient. It should be vertical and at the nurse's eye level.
- Ask the patient to refrain from talking or eating during the procedure, because this can result in an inaccurate higher BP (McAlister & Straus, 2001).
- Estimate the systolic pressure: palpate the brachial artery, inflate the cuff and note the reading when the brachial pulse disappears. Then deflate the cuff.

- Inflate the cuff to 30 mmHg above the estimated systolic level, which was required to occlude the brachial pulse. Approximately 5% of the population has an auscultatory gap; this is when the Korotkoff's sounds disappear just below the systolic pressure and reappear above the diastolic pressure (Talley & O'Connor, 2001). Estimating the systolic pressure will help ensure that the cuff is sufficiently inflated to record an accurate systolic pressure.
- Palpate the brachial artery.
- Place the diaphragm of the stethoscope gently over the brachial artery. Avoid applying excessive pressure on the diaphragm and do not tuck the diaphragm under the edge of the cuff, because either of these actions could partially occlude the brachial artery, delaying the occurrence of the Korotoff sounds (Dougherty & Lister, 2004).
- Open the valve and slowly deflate the cuff at a rate of 2–3 mm/s, recording when the Korotkoff sounds first appear (systolic) and disappear (diastolic).
- Document the systolic and diastolic BP readings on the patient's observation chart following local protocols. Compare with previous readings and inform nurse in charge/medical team as appropriate.

(Sources: British Hypertensive Society 2006a and 2006b, NICE & British Hypertensive Society, 2006 and Jevon 2007)

Errors in blood pressure measurement
Errors in BP measurement can occur for several reasons, including:

- Defective equipment, e.g. leaking tubing or a faulty valve
- Failure to ensure the mercury column reads 0 mmHg at rest
- Too rapid deflation of the cuff
- Use of incorrectly sized cuff: if it is too small the BP will be overestimated and if it is too big the blood pressure will be underestimated
- Cuff not at the same level as the heart

- Failure to observe the mercury level properly – the top of the mercury column should be at eye level
- Poor technique (e.g. failing to note when the sounds disappear)
- Digit preference, rounding the reading up to the nearest 5 or 10 mmHg
- Observer bias, e.g. expecting a young patient's BP to be normal.

(Source: British Hypertensive Society (2006a)

Automated blood pressure devices

When automated BP devices (Figure 4.2) were first manufactured, their accuracy and reliability were questioned (Beevers *et al.*, 2001). However, improved technology has led to the development of more accurate and reliable devices (Beevers *et al.*, 2001), some of which have been tested and approved for use by the British Hypertensive Society (2006a).

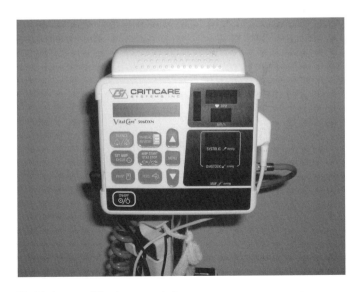

Fig 4.2 Automated blood pressure device

Most automated devices measure BP using one of the following techniques:

- Oscillometry to detect arterial blood flow (most commonly used device)
- A microphone to detect the Korotkoff sounds
- Ultrasound to detect arterial blood flow.

(British Hypertensive Society, 2006a)

Procedure for automated measurement of blood pressure

The principles for the accurate measurement of BP using an automated electronic device will be similar to the manual recording of BP using a sphygmomanometer in respect of patient preparation, patient position and cuff choice/placement (Dougherty & Lister, 2004). However, when using an automated electronic device, it is important to be familiar with its working and to follow the manufacturer's recommendations when using it.

DEFINITION OF HYPOTENSION

Hypotension is when the BP is abnormally low (McFerran & Martin, 2003). It is not possible to define hypotension at a particular level of BP because it depends upon the patient's clinical condition and pre-morbid state, e.g. history of chronic hypertension (Adam & Osborne, 2005). In addition, BP readings must be placed in the context of what is normal for that individual patient, e.g. a BP of 90/60 may be well tolerated and indeed normal in a fit young adult (Gwinnutt, 2006).

However, in practical terms, if the systolic BP is < 90 mmHg, this is generally considered to be hypotension (Wyatt *et al.*, 2006). This is reflected in many early warning scoring systems (Goldhill *et al.*, 1999 and Hodgetts *et al.*, 2004).

CAUSES OF HYPOTENSION

Causes of hypotension include:

- *Hypovolaemia*: e.g. dehydration/inadequate intake of fluid, haemorrhage, severe vomiting/diarrhoea, severe burns

- *Cardiogenic*: e.g. myocardial infarction, cardiogenic shock, cardiac arrhythmias and cardiomyopathy
- *Sepsis*
- *Anaphylaxis*
- *Drugs*: e.g. opiates, β-blockers
- *Spinal shock*
- *Pulmonary embolism.*

PHYSIOLOGY OF HYPOTENSION

Blood pressure is determined by cardiac output and vascular resistance (Waugh & Grant, 2006). Hypotension can therefore only result from a fall in cardiac output, a fall in vascular resistance or a fall in both (Smith, 2003). To understand the physiology of hypotension, it is helpful to understand what can lead to a fall in cardiac output and vascular resistance.

Cardiac output

Cardiac output can be defined as the amount of blood ejected from the left ventricle in 1 min (Adam & Osborne, 2005). The amount of blood expelled by each contraction is defined as the stroke volume. In a healthy adult at rest, the stroke volume is approximately 70 ml and the heart rate is 72 bpm: therefore the cardiac output at rest will be approximately 5 l/min (70 × 72) (Waugh & Grant, 2006).

Cardiac output is determined by heart rate, preload, myocardial contractility and afterload (Myburgh, 2004):

- *Heart rate*: bradycardia can lead to a reduction in cardiac output; in tachycardia, reduced diastolic filling time can again lead to a fall in cardiac output.
- *Preload*: the tension of the myocardial fibres at the end of diastole just before ventricular contraction (Hinds & Watson 1996). Starling's law of the heart states that 'the force of myocardial contraction is directly proportional to the initial fibre length', i.e. stretched fibres contract more forcefully (not over-stretched)

(Jevon & Ewens, 2007). Venous return is the main factor determining preload and as the filling pressure falls, cardiac output falls. Hypovolaemia will lead to a reduced preload and a consequent reduction in cardiac output.

- *Myocardial contractility*: the ability of the heart to function independently of changes in preload and afterload (Hinds & Watson 1996). It is commonly referred to as the 'force of contraction'. A reduction in contractility will lead to a fall in cardiac output (Smith, 2003). Factors affecting myocardial contractility include myocardial infarction, pulmonary embolism and myocardial depression due to sepsis (Ahern & Philpott, 2002).
- *Afterload*: the resistance to the outflow of blood provided by the vasculature, which must be overcome by the ventricles during contraction. In the clinical setting a rise in afterload, particularly in the failing heart, results in a decrease in cardiac output (Lee & Branch 1997).

Peripheral resistance

Peripheral resistance is the resistance to the flow of blood determined by the tone of the vascular musculature and the diameter of the blood vessels (Mosby, 1998). The smooth muscle in the arterioles is controlled by the vasomotor centre in the medulla. It is in a state of partial contraction caused by continuous sympathetic nerve activity, often referred to as 'sympathetic tone'.

A rise in peripheral resistance will lead to a fall in cardiac output because there is increased resistance to cardiac emptying; this is a rare primary cause of hypotension (Smith, 2003). A fall in peripheral resistance can also lead to hypotension; causes include sepsis, drug overdoses, damage to the upper spinal cord and epidural analgesia with local anaesthetic agents (Smith, 2003).

ADVERSE EFFECTS OF HYPOTENSION

Hypotension leads to poor perfusion of the vital organs. Adverse effects of hypotension include:

- *Renal system*: decreased renal perfusion leads to a fall in the glomerular filtration rate and oliguria; acute renal failure could develop
- *Brain*: reduced cerebral perfusion can lead to lightheadedness, drowsiness, confusion, agitation, syncope and coma
- *Heart*: decreased coronary perfusion can lead to myocardial ischaemia and infarction
- *Gut*: decreased gut perfusion can lead to bowel ischaemia
- *Skin*: poor skin perfusion will lead to pallor and cool peripheries; digital ischaemia could develop.

(Sources: Smith, 2003 and Adam & Osborne, 2005)

CIRCULATORY SHOCK

Circulatory shock can be defined as acute circulatory failure with inadequate or inappropriately distributed tissue perfusion resulting in generalized cellular hypoxia (Graham & Parke, 2005). A complex physiological phenomenon, shock is a life-threatening condition with a variety of causes. Without treatment it leads to cell starvation, cell death, organ dysfunction, organ failure and eventually death (Collins, 2000, Hand, 2001). The presence of shock is best detected by looking for signs of compromised end-organ perfusion (Graham & Parke, 2005).

Classification of circulatory shock

Shock can be defined as acute circulatory failure with inadequate or inappropriately distributed tissue perfusion resulting in generalized cellular hypoxia (Graham & Parke, 2005). Hypotension is often a late sign of shock (Smith, 2003).

There are four major classifications of shock: cardiogenic, hypovolaemic, distributive and obstructive (Bridges & Dukes, 2005):

- *Hypovolaemic shock*: although the heart may be pumping effectively, loss of circulating volume results in a low perfusion state (Collins, 2000) and reduced O_2 delivery. Causes of hypovolaemia are either from internal fluid shifts or external fluid losses (Diehl-Oplinger & Kaminski, 2004). Causes of internal fluid shift from intravascular compartments to 'third space' (intra-cellular or extracellular) compartments include intestinal obstruction, pancreatitis and peritonitis (Collins, 2000 and Diehl-Oplinger & Kaminski, 2004). Causes of external fluid loss include haemorrhage, burns, severe diarrhoea and vomiting (Hand, 2001).

- *Cardiogenic shock*: caused by severe heart failure (Leach, 2004) usually secondary to acute myocardial infarction (AMI), but can also complicate cardiomyopathy, trauma or a cardiac arrhythmia.
- *Distributive shock*: arises from abnormality of the peripheral circulation and can be divided into three different types: septic, anaphylactic and neurogenic shock (Hand, 2001). In septic and anaphylactic shock, the capillaries become permeable, leading to fluid leakage from the vasculature to the interstitial space. In neurogenic shock, damage to the spinal cord or brain stem, emotional trauma or drugs cause a reduction in sympathetic activity, resulting in massive vasodilation (Collins, 2000).
- *Obstructive shock*: caused by circulatory obstruction (Leach, 2004). Causes include pulmonary embolism, tension pneumo-thorax and cardiac tamponade.

Failure of oxygen supply to meet metabolic needs is the feature common to all forms of circulatory failure or 'shock': prevention, early identification and correction of tissue hypoxia are therefore necessary skills in managing the critically ill patient (Leach & Treacher, 2002). Prompt, effective treatment of 'early' shock may prevent progression to 'late' shock and organ failure (Leach & Treacher, 2002). Therefore, once hypotension is detected, rapid, effective treatment should be started and the cause identified (Smith, 2003).

TREATMENT OF HYPOTENSION

Hypotension should be considered a medical emergency (Smith, 2003). The main aim of initial treatment is to buy time to stabilize the patient's condition so that a more definitive diagnosis can be made and more expert help can be arranged (Gwinnutt, 2006). The key objectives of the management of hypotension are to:

- Identify and treat the underlying cause
- Maintain tissue oxygenation by ensuring adequate cardiac output and adequate arterial oxygen saturation
- Maintain tissue perfusion pressures by increasing systemic BP.

(Adam & Osborne, 2005)

Senior help should be requested and investigations/treatment should occur simultaneously (Wyatt *et al.*, 2006). If the hypotension is considered to be drug induced, e.g. nitrate infusion, β-blockers, stop the offending drug and seek medical advice. The following treatment action plan is recommended:

- Ensure the patient has a clear airway and is breathing adequately, and administer high concentration oxygen: use a mask with a non-rebreathe bag and high-flow oxygen (15l/min).
- Consider nursing the patient in a supine position; it may be necessary to raise his legs (Resuscitation Council UK, 2006).
- Attach pulse oximeter. If peripheral perfusion is poor, it may not detect a pulsatile flow or provide an oxygen saturation reading (Smith, 2003).
- Attach a cardiac monitor and monitor the ECG.
- Insert one or more large (14 or 16 G) (Figure 4.3) IV cannulae (use short, wide-bore cannulae, as they have the highest flow rate) (Resuscitation Council UK, 2005).
- Take blood from the cannula for full blood count, urea and electrolytes, glucose, liver function tests, lactate and coagulation screen (Wyatt *et al.*, 2006). Blood cultures and cross-matching may also be necessary. If haemorrhage is severe, request type specific blood. If haemorrhage is life threatening, request up to 4 units of O negative blood (Figure 4.4) (Hodgetts *et al.*, 2004). Ideally this should be cross matched or at least type specific, although sometimes the urgency of the situation will dictate otherwise.

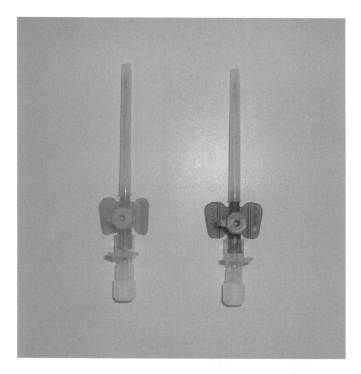

Fig 4.3 Wide bore IV cannulae

- Administer a rapid fluid challenge (over 5–10 min) of 1 l of warmed crystalloid solution (Resuscitation Council UK, 2005), e.g. 0.9% normal saline. Patients with severe hypotension due to cardiac failure may not tolerate such a rapid and large fluid bolus (Gwinnutt, 2006). Exercise caution with i.v. fluid administration in these patients (Wyatt *et al.*, 2006); administer i.v. fluids more slowly and use smaller volumes of fluid (250 ml) (Gwinnutt, 2006) and closely monitor these patients, e.g. auscultate the chest for crepitations after each bolus, consider a central venous pressure (CVP) line and CVP monitoring

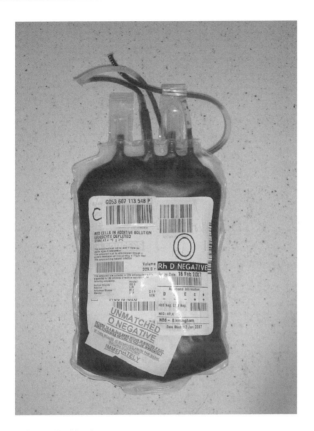

Fig 4.4 O negative blood

(Resuscitation Council UK, 2005). If signs and symptoms of cardiac failure occur (e.g. dyspnoea, increased heart rate and pulmonary crepitations on auscultation), decrease the fluid infusion rate or stop the fluids altogether; alternative methods of improving tissue perfusion include inotropic or vasopressor drugs (Resuscitation Council UK, 2005).

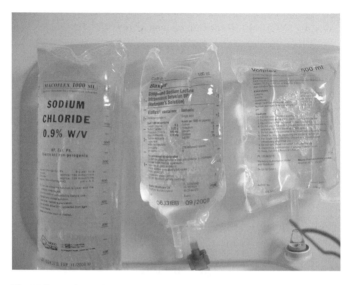

Fig 4.5 Resuscitation fluids for hypotension

- Reassess the patient's pulse rate and BP every 5 min: the target is the patient's normal BP or, if this is unknown, or a BP >100 mmHg systolic (Resuscitation Council UK, 2005). As the BP improves, the patient's clinical condition should also improve, e.g. heart rate slowing (caution!), signs of improved perfusion such as improved consciousness level, skin colour and urine output.
- Administer further i.v. fluids (Figure 4.5) if the patient shows no signs of improvement.
- Insert a urinary catheter and monitor urine output
- Consider vasoactive drugs if fluids alone fail to correct the hypotension (Smith, 2003). Vasoactive drugs include adrenaline and noradrenaline.
- Identify and treat the specific cause of the hypotension; specific treatments are detailed in Box 4.1.

Box 4.1 Treatment of specific causes of hypotension

Myocardial infarction: thrombolysis/angioplasty
Pulmonary embolism: thrombolysis
Drugs/poisons: specific antidotes
Sepsis: antibiotics
Anaphylaxis: adrenaline
Haemorrhage: surgery
Bradycardia: atropine/pacing (see Chapter 6)
Tachyarrhythmia: specific anti-arrhythmic therapy (see Chapter 6)
                                   (Sources: Jevon, 2002 and Wyatt *et al.*, 2006)

CONCLUSION

Hypotension, a sign that the patient is in shock, is common in the critically ill patient. It should be regarded as a medical emergency, requiring rapid treatment and identification of the cause. Failure to treat it effectively could lead to poor perfusion of the vital organs. It is commonly caused by hypovolaemia, which generally responds well to fluid resuscitation. In this chapter the treatment of hypotension has been described.

REFERENCES

Adam, S, & Osborne, S. (2005) *Critical Care Nursing Science and Practice,* 2nd edn. Oxford University Press, Oxford.

Ahern, J, & Philpot, P. (2002) Assessing acutely ill patients on general wards. *Nursing Standard* **16,** 47–55.

Beevers, G, Lip, G, O'Brien, E. (2001) *ABC of Hypertension,* 4th edn. BMJ Books, London.

Berger, A. (2001) How does it work? Oscillatory blood pressure monitoring devices. *BMJ* **323,** 9–19.

British Hypertensive Society (2006a) *Let's Do It Well.* www.bhsoc. org/pdfs/hit.pdf

British Hypertensive Society (2006a) *Let's Do It Well.* www.bhsoc. org/pdfs/hit.pdf

British Hypertensive Society (2006b) Blood Pressure Measurement with Mercury Blood Pressure Monitors. www.bhsoc.org

Department of Health (2000). *National Service Framework for Coronary Heart Disease*. Department of Health, London.

Dougherty, L, & Lister, S. (2004) *The Royal Marsden Hospital Manual of Clinical Nursing Procedures*, 6th edn. Blackwell Publishing, Oxford.

Ford, M, Hennessey, I, Japp, A. (2005) *Introduction to Clinical Examination*. Elsvier, Edinburgh.

Goldhill, D, *et al.* (1999) Physiological values and procedures in the 24 hours before ICU admission from the ward. *Anaesthesia* **54,** 529–534.

Graham, C, & Parke, T. (2005) Critical care in the emergency department: shock and circulatory support. *Emerg Med J* **22,** 17–21.

Hill, M, & Grim, C. (1991) How to take a precise blood pressure. *Am J Nurs* **91,** 38–42.

Gwinnutt, C. (2006) *Clinical Anaesthesia*, 2nd edn. Blackwell Publishing, Oxford.

Hodgetts, T, Ineson, N, Shaikh, L *et al.* (2004) *In-Hospital Cardiac Arrest: Treatment Guidelines* www.metproject.org.uk

Jevon, P, & Ewens, B. (2007) *Monitoring the Critically Ill Patient,* 2nd edn. Blackwell Publishing, Oxford.

Jones, A, Yiannibas, V, Johnson, C, Kline, J. (2006) Emergency department hypotension predicts sudden unexpected in-hospital mortality: a prospective cohort study. *Chest* **130,** 941–946.

Marieb, E. (2001) *Human Anatomy & Physiology*. Benjamin Cummings, San Francisco.

McAlister, F, & Straus, S. (2001) Evidence based treatment for hypertension – measurement of blood pressure: an evidence based review. *BMJ* **322,** 908–911.

McFerran, T, & Martin, E. (2003) *Minidictionary for Nurses*. Oxford University Press, Oxford.

MHRA (2005) *Report of the Independent Advisory Group on Blood Pressure Monitoring in Clinical Practice*. MRHA, London.

Mosby (2006) *Mosby's Medical Dictionary*, 7th edn. Mosby, St Louis.

NICE & the British Hypertensive Society (2006) *NICE/BHS Hypertension Guideline Review*. 28 June 2006 www.bhsoc.org/NICE_BHS_Guidelines.stm

Resuscitation Council (UK) (2005) *Resuscitation Guidelines 2005.* Resuscitation Council (UK), London.

Resuscitation Council (UK) (2006) *Advanced Life Support,* 5th edn. Resuscitation Council (UK), London.

Smith, G. (2003) *ALERT Acute Life-Threatening Events Recognition and Treatment,* 2nd edn. University of Portsmouth, Portsmouth.

Talley, N, & O'Connor, S. (2001) *Clinical Examination: A Systematic Guide to Physical Diagnosis.* Blackwell Science, Oxford.

Waugh, A, & Grant, A. (2006) *Ross and Wilson Anatomy and Physiology in Health and Illness,* 10th edn. Churchill Livingstone, Edinburgh.

Wyatt, J, Illingworth, R, Graham, C *et al.* (2006) *Oxford Handbook of Emergency Medicine,* 3rd edn. Oxford University Press, Oxford.

5 | Treating a Patient with Bradycardia or Tachycardia

INTRODUCTION

A successful strategy to reduce the mortality and morbidity of cardiac arrest must include appropriate treatment to prevent potentially serious cardiac arrhythmias and optimal treatment should they occur (Nolan *et al.*, 2005). If the patient has a brady-cardia or a tachycardia, effective management will be required. Generally, a bradycardia can be defined as a heart rate < 60 bpm and a tachycardia can be defined as a heart rate > 100 bpm (Resuscitation Council UK, 2006).

The Resuscitation Council (UK) provides guidance for the effective and safe management of the patient with a bradycardia (Figure 5.1) or tachycardia (a tachyarrhythmia, i.e. fast atrial fibrillation, narrow complex tachycardia and broad complex tachycardia, but not sinus tachycardia) (Figure 5.2) (Resuscitation Council UK, 2006). When determining the most appropriate management, it is paramount to assess the clinical condition of the patient and to ascertain whether the arrhythmia is life threatening or has the potential to deteriorate and become life threatening.

It must be stressed that sinus tachycardia, a common finding in the critically ill patient, is often a compensatory mechanism and treatment is aimed at correcting the underlying cause, e.g. hypovolaemia. The Resuscitation Council UK tachy-cardia algorithm (Figure 5.2) therefore does not apply to sinus tachycardia.

The aim of this chapter is to help the reader understand the treatment of a patient with a bradycardia or a tachycardia.

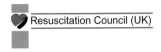 Resuscitation Council (UK)

Bradycardia Algorithm
(includes rates inappropriately slow for haemodynamic state)

If appropriate, give oxygen, cannulate a vein, and record a 12-lead ECG

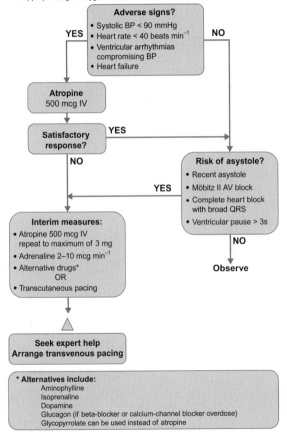

Adverse signs?
- Systolic BP < 90 mmHg
- Heart rate < 40 beats min^{-1}
- Ventricular arrhythmias compromising BP
- Heart failure

YES   NO

Atropine
500 mcg IV

Satisfactory response? YES

NO

Risk of asystole?
- Recent asystole
- Möbitz II AV block
- Complete heart block with broad QRS
- Ventricular pause > 3s

YES

NO

Interim measures:
- Atropine 500 mcg IV repeat to maximum of 3 mg
- Adrenaline 2–10 mcg min^{-1}
- Alternative drugs*
  OR
- Transcutaneous pacing

Observe

**Seek expert help
Arrange transvenous pacing**

* Alternatives include:
    Aminophylline
    Isoprenaline
    Dopamine
    Glucagon (if beta-blocker or calcium-channel blocker overdose)
    Glycopyrrolate can be used instead of atropine

Fig 5.1 Resuscitation Council (UK) bradycardia algorithm (Resuscitation Council UK)

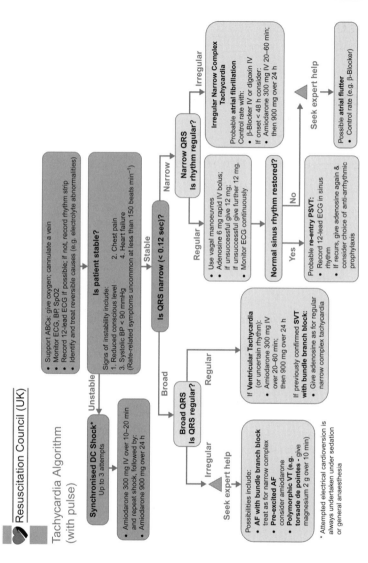

Fig 5.2 Resuscitation Council (UK) tachycardia algorithm (Resuscitation Council UK)

LEARNING OBJECTIVES

At the end of the chapter the reader will be able to:

❏ Discuss the management of sinus tachycardia
❏ List the causes of bradycardia and tachycardia
❏ Discuss the principles of the use of the bradycardia and tachy-cardia algorithms
❏ List the adverse clinical signs that may be associated with bradycardia and tachycardia
❏ Discuss the treatment of bradycardia
❏ Discuss the treatment of tachycardia.

MANAGEMENT OF SINUS TACHYCARDIA

Sinus tachycardia (Figure 5.3) is a common finding in the critically ill patient. It is not classed as a tachyarrhythmia; it is usually a response to another physiological or pathological state (Resuscitation Council UK, 2006).

Causes

Causes of sinus tachycardia include:

• Hypovolaemia
• Sepsis
• Heart failure
• Myocardial infarction
• Severe pain
• Anxiety
• Thyrotoxicosis.

(Jevon, 2002 and Gwinnutt, 2006)

ECG features

It is important to be able to recognize the ECG features of sinus tachycardia (Figure 5.3):

• Rate is >100 but generally <140 bpm
• Usually regular
• P waves present; P waves associated with QRS complexes

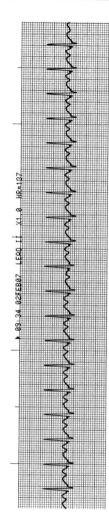

09:34 02FEB07 LEAD II X1.0 HR=137

Fig 5.3 Sinus tachycardia

- Non-paroxysmal, i.e. it does not start and end abruptly – a common finding in tachyarrhythmias.

Treatment

Treatment is aimed at the underlying cause, not the sinus tachycardia (Gwinnutt, 2006). The Resuscitation Council UK algorithm for the treatment of tachycardia (Figure 5.2) does not apply to sinus tachycardia.

CAUSES OF BRADYCARDIA AND TACHYCARDIA

Causes of bradycardia

Causes of a bradycardia include:

- Myocardial infarction
- Drugs, e.g. β-blockers, digoxin
- Hypothermia
- Hypoxia
- Hypothyroidism
- Hypovolaemia
- Raised intracranial pressure

(Jevon, 2002, Gwinnutt, 2006 and Wyatt *et al.*, 2006)

> Bradycardia may be a normal finding in a young fit adult (Gwinnutt, 2006).

Causes of tachycardia

Causes of tachycardia (fast atrial fibrillation, narrow complex tachycardia and broad complex tachycardia) include:

- Electrolyte abnormalities
- Myocardial ischaemia/infarction
- Drugs
- Thyrotoxicosis
- Cardiac disease.

PRINCIPLES OF THE USE OF THE BRADYCARDIA AND TACHYCARDIA ALGORITHMS

The Resuscitation Council (UK)'s algorithms for the management of bradycardia (Figure 5.1) and tachycardia (Figure 5.2) are designed for the non-specialist in order to provide effective and safe treatment in the emergency situation (Resuscitation Council UK, 2006). If the patient is not acutely ill, other treatment options may be considered and there is usually time to seek help from a senior clinician, e.g. cardiologist (Nolan *et al.*, 2005).

The following points regarding the use of the algorithms need to be emphasized:

- They are specifically designed for the emergency situation and are not intended to encompass all clinical situations (Colquhoun & Vincent, 1999)
- The arrows indicate progression from one stage of treatment to the next, but only if the cardiac arrhythmia persists
- Several variables will influence the treatment, including the cardiac arrhythmia, the haemodynamic status of the patient, local procedures and local circumstances/facilities/expertise
- The drug doses are based on average body weight; in some situations adjustments to the dose may be required
- Anti-arrhythmic strategies can be pro-arrhythmic
- Anti-arrhythmic drugs can cause adverse effects, e.g. amiodarone can cause hypotension
- Expert help must be summoned early if necessary.

(Sources: Jevon, 2002 and Nolan *et al.*, 2005)

The tachycardia algorithm (Figure 5.2) outlines the treatment of a tachyarrhythmia, i.e. fast atrial fibrillation, narrow complex tachycardia and broad complex tachycardia, but not sinus tachycardia (Resuscitation Council UK, 2006).

ADVERSE SIGNS

In the majority of patients, the presence of certain adverse signs or symptoms will determine whether treatment is indicated and the urgency with which it is required (Resuscitation Council UK,

2006). The following adverse signs indicate that the patient is unstable because of the arrhythmia.

- *Clinical evidence of low cardiac output*: pallor, sweating, cold and clammy extremities (increased sympathetic activity) and impaired consciousness level (e.g. drowsiness and confusion) due to reduced cerebral blood flow and hypotension (e.g. systolic blood pressure <90 mmHg) (Nolan *et al.*, 2005 and Resuscitation Council UK, 2006).
- *Excessive tachycardia (typically heart rate > 150 min)*: as diastole is shortened, the heart does not have sufficient time to fill properly, resulting in a fall in cardiac output (Resuscitation Council UK, 2006). In addition, the shortened diastole can lead to a fall in coronary blood flow (the majority of coronary blood flow occurs during diastole), which can lead to myocardial ischaemia and chest pain (Nolan *et al.*, 2005). Broad complex tachycardias are less well tolerated than narrow complex tachycardias (Resuscitation Council UK, 2006).
- *Excessive bradycardia (typically heart rate < 40)*: although this is usually defined as a heart rate < 40/min, higher rates may not be well tolerated by some patients with poor cardiac reserve (Colquhoun & Vincent, 1999).
- *Heart failure*: the efficiency of the myocardial pump action of the heart can become compromised, which can lead to heart failure. Left ventricular failure is manifested by breathlessness, pulmonary crackles on auscultation and pulmonary oedema on chest X-ray; right ventricular failure is manifested by peripheral oedema (leg oedema, raised jugular venous pressure and hepatic engorgement) (Resuscitation Council UK, 2006).
- *Chest pain*: if the patient has chest pain, this indicates that the cardiac arrhythmia is causing myocardial ischaemia. This is particular significant if the patient has existing coronary artery disease or structural heart disease, because it could cause further life-threatening complications, including cardiopulmonary arrest (Nolan *et al.*, 2005).

(Sources: Nolan *et al.*, 2005 and Resuscitation Council UK, 2006)

TREATMENT OF A BRADYCARDIA

Bradycardia will be a normal finding in some patients, particular those who are young and fit (Gwinnutt, 2006)

The emergency treatment of bradycardia (Figure 5.1) will depend upon two important clinical factors:

- The clinical condition of the patient and whether adverse signs are present?
- The risk of asystole (Wyatt *et al.*, 2006).
- Undertake rapid assessment of airway, breathing and circulation – ascertain whether any adverse signs are present.
- Administer high concentration oxygen and commence pulse oximetry.
- Secure i.v. access and commence ECG monitoring; establish that the patient has bradycardia (Figure 5.4).
- If the patient is hypotensive and is feeling light-headed, lie him flat with his legs raised.
- If adverse signs present (e.g. systolic blood pressure <90 mmHg, heart rate <40 bpm, altered consciousness level, heart failure) administer atropine 500 mg i.v.: this is the first drug of choice in a bradycardia (Wyatt *et al.*, 2006). The dose can be repeated every 3–5 min up to a maximum of 3 mg i.v. Care should be taken in patients with an acute coronary syndrome because the increase in heart rate may worsen the ischaemia.
- Establish if there is a risk of asystole. This is possible if there has been a recent episode of asystole or if either second-degree atrioventricular block Mobitz type 2 or third-degree atrioventricular block (complete heart block) (particularly if QRS complex is broad or if the initial rate is < 40/min) is present (Resuscitation Council UK, 2006).

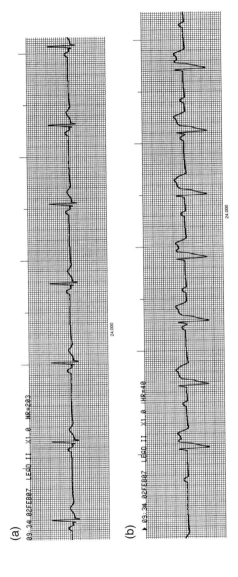

(a)

09:34 02FEB07 LEAD II X1.0 HR=203

(b)

▶ 09:34 02FEB07 LEAD II X1.0 HR=40

Fig 5.4 ECG example of bradycardia

- If there is no response to atropine and the patient remains unstable and/or there is a risk of asystole, ensure that appropriate help, e.g. a cardiologist, has been requested because pacing will usually be required (Nolan *et al.*, 2005). The definitive treatment will be transvenous pacing, but while awaiting the appropriate expertise and facilities to be arranged, interim measures to help prevent deterioration and improve the patient's condition include transcutaneous (external) pacing or fist pacing if this is not available, or an adrenaline infusion (Resuscitation Council UK, 2006).

Transcutaneous (external) pacing

Cardiac pacing is the delivery of a small electrical current to the heart to stimulate myocardial contraction. Transcutaneous or external pacing can be quickly and easily established and buys time for the spontaneous recovery of the conduction system or for more definitive treatment to be established, e.g. transvenous pacing. Transcutaneous pacing can be painful: analgesia and sedation may be required. The procedure for transcutaneous pacing is:

- If appropriate, explain the procedure to the patient.
- Ideally, first remove excess chest hair from the pacing electrode sites by clipping close to the patient's skin using a pair of scissors (shaving the skin is not recommended, as any nicks in the skin can lead to burns and pain during pacing) (Resuscitation Council UK, 2006).
- Attach the pacing electrodes following the manufacturer's instructions.
- *Pacing-only electrodes*: attach the anterior electrode on the left anterior chest, midway between the xiphoid process and the left nipple (V2-V3 ECG electrode position) and attach the posterior electrode below the left scapula, lateral to the spine and at the same level as the anterior electrode – this anterior/posterior configuration will ensure that the position of the electrodes does not interfere with defibrillation (Resuscitation

Council UK, 2006). ECG monitoring will usually need to be established if an older pacing system is used (Resuscitation Council UK, 2006).

- *Multifunctional electrodes (pacing and defibrillation)*: place the anterior electrode below the right clavicle and the lateral electrode in the mid-axillary line lateral to the left nipple (V6 ECG electrode position) – this anterior-lateral position is convenient during cardiopulmonary resuscitation (CPR) as chest compressions do not have to be interrupted (Resuscitation Council UK, 2006).
- Check that the pacing electrodes and connecting cables are applied following the manufacturer's recommendations: if they are reversed, pacing may either be ineffective or high capture thresholds may be required (Resuscitation Council UK, 2006).
- Adjust the ECG gain (size) accordingly. This will help ensure that the intrinsic QRS complexes are sensed.
- Select demand mode on the pacing unit on the defibrillator.
- Select an appropriate rate for external pacing, usually 60–90/min.
- Set the pacing current at the lowest level, turn on the pacemaker unit and while observing both the patient and the ECG, gradually increase the current until electrical capture occurs (QRS complexes following the pacing spike) (Jevon, 2002). Electrical capture usually occurs when the current delivered is in the range of 50–100 mA (Resuscitation Council UK, 2006).
- Check the patient's pulse. If he has a palpable pulse (mechanical capture), request expert help and prepare for transvenous pacing. If no pulse, start CPR. If there is good electrical capture, but no mechanical capture, this is indicative of a non-viable myocardium (Resuscitation Council UK, 2006). Note, there is no electrical hazard if in contact with the patient during pacing (Resuscitation Council UK, 2006).

Fist pacing

If atropine has been ineffective and transcutaneous pacing is not immediately available, fist pacing can be attempted if the patient is in ventricular standstill or has extreme bradycardia (Resuscitation Council UK, 2006). Using a clenched fist, administer serial rhythmic blows over the left lower edge of the sternum to pace the heart at a rate of approximately 50–70 bpm (Nolan *et al.*, 2005).

Adrenaline infusion

If an external pacemaker is not immediately available, an adrenaline infusion can be started as a temporary measure (Wyatt *et al.*, 2006). Administer adrenaline via a controlled infusion at 2–10 mg/min, titrating it according to the effect (add 6 mg of adrenaline to 500 ml 0.9% sodium chloride infused at a rate of 10–50 ml/h) (Wyatt *et al.*, 2006).

TREATMENT OF A TACHYCARDIA

The Resuscitation Council UK tachycardia algorithm (Figure 5.2) works on the basis that, irrespective of the exact underlying ECG rhythm, most of the initial treatment principles for a tachyarrhythmia are the same (Wyatt *et al.*, 2006).

- Rapid assessment of airway, breathing and circulation: assess for the presence of adverse signs, e.g. systolic blood pressure < 90 mmHg, heart rate >150 bpm, chest pain, heart failure and altered consciousness level, e.g. drowsiness, confusion (Resuscitation Council UK, 2006).
- While undertaking this assessment, ensure high concentration oxygen is commenced, appropriate monitoring is established (oxygen saturation and ECG) and i.v. access is secured.
- Establish that the patient has a tachycardia (Figure 5.5), taking care to ensure that it is not sinus tachycardia.
- If the patient is hypotensive or is feeling lightheaded, lie him flat.
- Ensure appropriate help is called.
- Record a single-lead ECG strip from the monitor.
- If possible, record a 12-lead ECG; this will help to establish the correct interpretation of the rhythm, either before treatment or

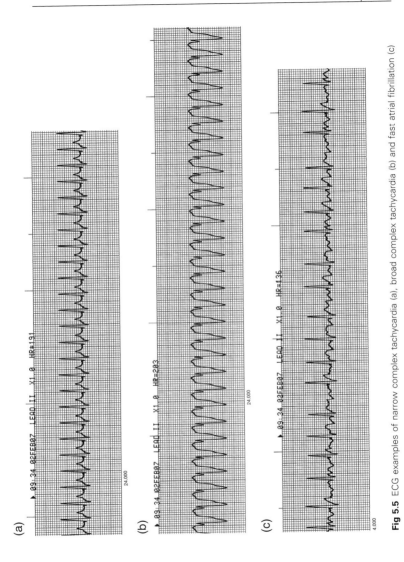

(a)

▶ 09:34 02FEB07 LEAD II X1.0 HR=191

24.000

(b)

▶ 09:34 02FEB07 LEAD II X1.0 HR=203

24.000

(c)

▶ 09:34 02FEB07 LEAD II X1.0 HR=136

4.000

Fig 5.5 ECG examples of narrow complex tachycardia (a), broad complex tachycardia (b) and fast atrial fibrillation (c)

retrospectively if necessary with the help of an expert (Nolan *et al.*, 2005).

- Identify and treat any underlying causes, e.g. electrolyte abnormalities, particularly hypokalaemia.
- If the patient is unstable (e.g. altered consciousness level, systolic blood pressure < 90 mmHg, chest pain, heart failure), prepare for synchronized electrical cardioversion (see below).
- If the patient is stable, treatment will depend on whether the rhythm is regular or irregular and whether the QRS complex is narrow (< 0.12 s or three small squares) or broad (0.12 s or more); treatment options initially include vagal manoeuvres and anti-arrhythmic drugs (see below).
- Once the arrhythmia has been successfully treated, repeat the 12-lead ECG to enable detection of any underlying abnormalities that may require long-term therapy (Nolan *et al.*, 2005).

Vagal manoeuvres

These are used to stimulate the vagus nerve and induce a reflex slowing of the heart (Smith, 2003). They are successful in terminating 25% of narrow complex tachycardias (Resuscitation Council UK, 2000).

Caution should be exercised regarding the use of vagal manoeuvres. Profound vagal tone can induce sudden bradycardia and trigger ventricular fibrillation, particularly in the presence of digitalis toxicity or acute cardiac ischaemia (Colquhoun & Vincent, 1999).

The most commonly used vagal manoeuvres are:

- *Carotid sinus massage*: should not be used in the presence of a carotid bruit as atheromatous plaque rupture could embolize into the cerebral circulation causing a cerebral vascular accident; elderly patients are more vulnerable to plaque rupture and cerebral vascular complications (Skinner & Vincent, 1997).
- *Valsalva manoeuvre*: forced expiration against a closed glottis, e.g. ask the patient to blow into a 20-ml syringe with enough

force to push the plunger back (Resuscitation Council UK, 2006).

Anti-arrhythmic drugs

As anti-arrhythmic drug therapy has a slower onset of action and is less reliable than electrical cardioversion in converting a tachycardia to a normal sinus rhythm, drugs are generally reserved for stable patients without adverse signs and electrical cardioversion is used in unstable patients displaying adverse signs (Nolan *et al.*, 2005).

> All anti-arrhythmic treatments can be pro-arrhythmic, i.e. clinical deterioration of the patient may be due to the treatment rather than lack of effect (Nolan *et al.*, 2005).

Adenosine

Very effective at terminating tachyarrhythmias that originate in the atrioventricular junction (Nolan *et al.*, 2005). As its half-life is very short (approximately 10–15 s), it should be administered as a rapid i.v. bolus followed by a flush. The recommended initial dose is 6 mg; two further doses of 12 mg may be administered if required (Resuscitation Council UK, 2006). During administration, record an ECG rhythm strip and warn the patient that he may experience flushing and chest pain (Wyatt *et al.*, 2006).

Amiodarone

Widely used for the management of tachyarrhythmias. The standard dose is 300 mg i.v. over 10–60 min (depending on the circumstances and haemodynamic stability of the patient) followed by an infusion of 900 mg over 24 h (Nolan *et al.*, 2005). As it cannot be mixed with normal saline, 5% dextrose is usually used as a diluting solution. It is important to monitor the patient for adverse effects including hypotension and bradycardia. As amiodarone can cause thrombophlebitis, it should ideally be administered through a central vein.

Verapamil

Occasionally used for narrow complex tachycardia. The initial dose of verapamil is 2.5–5 mg i.v. over 2 min; repeated doses may be necessary (Nolan *et al.*, 2005).

Synchronized electrical cardioversion

Synchronized electrical cardioversion is the delivery of a shock to the myocardium to terminate a tachyarrhythmia. It is indicated if the patient has a tachyarrhythmia and is unstable and compromised, e.g. impaired consciousness level, chest pain, heart failure, hypotension or other signs of shock (Nolan *et al.*, 2005). It can also be considered if chemical (drug) therapy is ineffective.

The shock must be delivered with the R wave and not the T wave (Deakin & Nolan, 2005), as delivery of the shock during the refractory period of the cardiac cycle (T wave) could induce ventricular fibrillation (Lown, 1967). The defibrillator must therefore be synchronized with the patient's ECG.

For synchronized electrical cardioversion of a broad complex tachycardia and atrial fibrillation, 120–150 J biphasic (200 J monophasic) is recommended initially; and for a regular narrow complex tachycardia or atrial flutter (lower energy levels are usually successful) 70–120 J biphasic (100 J monophasic) is recommended initially (Resuscitation Council UK, 2005). As biphasic waveforms are more effective than monophasic waveforms for cardioversion of atrial fibrillation, a biphasic defibrillator should ideally be used (Deakin & Nolan, 2005).

Due to risk of a cerebral embolism arising from stasis of blood in the left atrium, a patient with atrial fibrillation > 48 h should normally not receive electrical synchronized cardioversion until he has been fully anti-coagulated or transoesophageal echocardiography has confirmed the absence of an atrial clot (Resuscitation Council UK, 2006).

The following procedure is recommended for synchronized electrical cardioversion:

- If possible record a 12-lead ECG.
- Explain the procedure to the patient. Consent should be obtained if possible. If the patient is conscious, he must be anaesthetized or sedated for the procedure (Nolan *et al.*, 2005). This usually involves requesting the help of an anaesthetist.
- Ensure the resuscitation equipment is immediately at hand.
- Establish ECG monitoring using the defibrillator, which is going to be used for cardioversion.
- Select a monitoring lead that provides a clear ECG trace on the monitor, e.g. lead II.
- Press the 'synch' button on the defibrillator (Figure 5.6a).
- Check the ECG trace to ensure that only the R waves are being synchronized; i.e. a 'synchronized dot or arrow' should appear on each R wave (Figure 5.6b) and not on any other parts of the ECG complex, e.g. tall T waves.
- Apply defibrillation gel pads to the patient's chest, one just to the right of the sternum, below the right clavicle, and the other in the mid-axillary line, approximately level with V6 ECG electrode or female breast (Deakin & Nolan, 2005).
- Select the appropriate energy level (see above) on the defibrillator.
- Place the defibrillator paddles firmly on the defibrillation pads. It is not necessary to apply the paddles according to their namesakes, i.e. sternum to sternum and apex to apex (Deakin & Nolan, 2005).
- Charge the defibrillator and shout 'stand clear'.
- Perform a visual sweep to ensure that all personnel are clear and that oxygen has been removed.
- Check the ECG monitor to ensure that the patient is still in the tachyarrhythmia that requires cardioversion, that the synchronized button is still activated and that it is still synchronizing with the R waves.
- Press both discharge buttons simultaneously to discharge the shock. There is usually a slight delay between pressing the shock buttons and shock discharge.

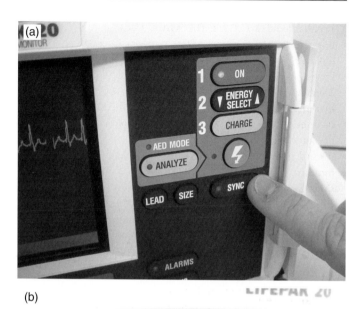

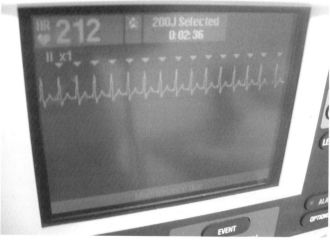

Fig 5.6a Synchronization: press the 'synch' button on the defibrillator
Fig 5.6b Check the ECG trace to ensure that only the R waves are being synchronized

- Re-assess the ECG trace. The 'synch' button will usually need to be reactivated if further cardioversion is required (on some defibrillators it is necessary to actually switch off the 'synch' button if further cardioversion is not indicated). Stepwise increases in energy will be required if cardioversion needs to be repeated (Deakin & Nolan, 2005). Amiodarone is indicated if three attempts at cardioversion have been unsuccessful (Nolan *et al.*, 2005).
- Record post successful cardioversion 12-lead ECG.
- Monitor the patient's vital signs until full recovery from anaesthetic or sedative.
- Ensure accurate documentation of the procedure.

CONCLUSION

If the patient has a bradycardia or tachycardia, effective management will be required. The Resuscitation Council (UK) provides guidance for the effective and safe management of these patients. When determining the most appropriate management, it is paramount to assess the clinical condition of the patient and to ascertain whether he is displaying adverse signs or not.

It must be stressed that sinus tachycardia, a common finding in the critically ill patient, is often a compensatory mechanism and treatment is aimed at correcting the underlying cause.

REFERENCES

Boodhoo, L, Bordoli, G, Mitchell, A *et al.* (2004) The safety and effectiveness of a nurse led cardioversion service under sedation. *Heart* **90,** 1443–1446.

Colquhoun, M, & Vincent, R. (1999) Management of peri-arrest arrhythmias. In: Colquhoun, M, Handley, A, Evans, T, eds. *ABC of Resuscitation*, 4th edn. BMJ Books, London.

Deakin, C, & Nolan J. (2005) European Resuscitation Council Guidelines for Resuscitation 2005: Section 3. Electrical therapies: automated external defibrillators, defibrillation, cardioversion and pacing. *Resuscitation* **675S,** S25–37.

Gwinnutt, C. (2006) *Clinical Anaesthesia,* 2nd edn. Blackwell Publishing, Oxford.

Jevon, P. (2001) *Advanced Cardiac Life Support.* Butterworth Heinemann, Oxford.

Lown, B. (1967) Electrical reversion of cardiac arrhythmias. *Br Heart J* **29,** 469–489.

Nolan, J, Deakin, C, Soar, J et al. (2005) European Resuscitation Council Guidelines for Resuscitation 2005: Section 4. Adult advanced life support. *Resuscitation* **675S,** S39–S86.

Page, R, Kerber, R, Russell J et al. (2002) Biphasic versus monophasic shock waveform for cardioversion of atrial fibrillation: the results of an international randomised, double-blinded multi-center trial. *J Am Coll Cardiol* **39,** 1956–1963.

Resuscitation Council (UK) (2006) *Advanced Life Support,* 5th edn. Resuscitation Council (UK), London.

Resuscitation Council (UK) (2005) *Resuscitation Guidelines 2005.* Resuscitation Council (UK), London.

Skinner, D, & Vincent, R. (1997) *Cardiopulmonary Resuscitation,* 2nd edn. Oxford University Press, Oxford.

Smith, G. (2003) *ALERT Acute Life-Threatening Events Recognition and Treatment,* 2nd edn. University of Portsmouth.

Wyatt, J, Illingworth, R, Graham, C et al. (2006) *Oxford Handbook of Emergency Medicine,* 3rd edn. Oxford University Press, Oxford.

Treating a Patient with Altered Consciousness Level

6

INTRODUCTION

Altered consciousness level is common in the critically ill patient and is associated with potentially life-threatening airway compromise. As a problem with airway, breathing or circulation can lead to altered consciousness level, the initial priorities are to ensure a clear airway, adequate breathing and adequate circulation. Identifying and, where possible, treating the underlying cause of altered consciousness is paramount.

The aim of this chapter is to understand the treatment of a patient with altered consciousness level.

LEARNING OBJECTIVES

At the end of this chapter the reader will be able to:

❏ Define level of consciousness
❏ List the common causes of altered consciousness level
❏ Outline the assessment of consciousness level
❏ Discuss the treatment of a patient with altered consciousness level.

DEFINITION OF LEVEL OF CONSCIOUSNESS

The patient's level of consciousness has been described as the degree of his arousal and awareness (Geraghty, 2005). It is dependent upon the interaction of the ascending reticular activating system situated in the brainstem and the cerebral hemispheres. Any disruption in this communication process will result in altered consciousness (Bassett & Makin, 2000).

The manifestation of altered consciousness implies an underlying brain dysfunction (Geraghty, 2005). Definitions of impaired consciousness are listed in Table 6.1.

COMMON CAUSES OF ALTERED CONSCIOUSNESS LEVEL

The onset of altered consciousness level may be sudden, e.g. following an acute head injury, or it may be gradual, for example, with the onset of poisoning or a deranged metabolism, as in hypoxia or hypoglycaemia (Geraghty, 2005).

Common causes of altered consciousness level include:

- Profound hypoxaemia
- Hypercapnia
- Cerebral hypoperfusion
- Recent administration of sedatives or analgesic drugs
- Hypoglycaemia
- Drug overdose
- Stroke
- Subarachnoid haemorrhage

Table 6.1 Definitions of impaired consciousness

Condition	Definition
Consciousness	Awareness of self and environment
Confusion	Reduced awareness, disorientation
Delirium	Disorientation, fear, irritability, misperception, hallucination
Obtundation	Reduced alertness, psychomotor retardation, drowsiness
Stupor	Unresponsiveness with arousal only by vigorous and repeated stimuli
Coma	Unarousable unresponsiveness
Vegetative state	Prolonged coma (>1month), some preservation of brainstem and motor reflexes
Akinetic mutism	Prolonged coma with apparent alertness and flaccid motor tone
Locked-in state	Total paralysis below third cranial nerve nuclei; normal or impaired mental function

(Reproduced with kind permission of Butterworth-Heinemann from Myburgh & Ohe, 1997)

- Convulsions
- Alcohol intoxication

(Sources: Wyatt *et al.*, 2006 and
Resuscitation Council UK, 2006)

ASSESSMENT OF CONSCIOUSNESS LEVEL

A variety of scales have been designed to assess consciousness level (Geraghty, 2005). It is not possible to measure consciousness level directly; it can be assessed only by observing the patient's behavioural response to different stimuli (Waterhouse, 2005).

During the initial rapid assessment of the critically ill patient it is helpful to use the AVPU scale, together with an examination of the pupils, to determine the patient's consciousness level. The Glasgow Coma Scale (GCS) should be used in the later full patient assessment to provide a more specific measurement of consciousness level (Smith, 2003). The National Institute for Health and Clinical Excellence (NICE) recommends the use of the GCS to assess all patients with head injuries (NICE, 2003).

AVPU

The AVPU scale is a quick and easy method to assess level of consciousness. It is ideal in the initial rapid ABCDE assessment of the critically ill patient:

- **A**lert
- Responds to **v**oice
- Responds to **p**ain
- **U**nconscious

(Resuscitation Council UK, 2006)

Examination of the pupils

Changes in the size, equality and reactivity of the pupils can provide important diagnostic information in the critically ill patient (Smith, 2003). Although not part of the GCS, examination of the pupils is an essential adjunct to it, especially when the patient's consciousness level is impaired (Berston *et al.*, 2003).

Pupillary reaction is an assessment of the third cranial nerve (oculomotor nerve), which controls constriction of the pupil. Compression of this nerve will result in fixed dilated pupils (Fairley, 2005). Any changes in pupil reaction, size or shape, together with other neurological signs, are an indication of raised intracranial pressure (ICP) and compression of the optic nerve (Mooney & Comerford, 2003).

Prior to undertaking pupillary assessment, the following should be noted:

- Any pre-existing irregularity with the pupils, e.g. cataracts, false eye and previous eye injury.
- Factors that cause pupillary dilation, e.g. medications including tricyclics, atropine and sympathomimetics and traumatic mydriasis (Bersten *et al.*, 2003)
- Factors that cause pupillary constriction, e.g. medications including narcotics (Fairley, 2005) and topical β-blockers.

Pupillary assessment should include the following observations.

- *Size (mm)*: prior to shining light into the eyes, estimate pupil size using the scale printed on the neurological assessment chart as a comparison. The average size is 2–5mm (Bersten *et al.*, 2003). Both pupils should be equal in size.
- *Shape*: should be round; abnormal shapes may indicate cerebral damage; oval shape could indicate intracranial hypertension (Fairley, 2005).
- *Reactivity to light*: a bright light source (usually a pen torch) should be moved from the outer aspect of the eye towards the pupil – a brisk constriction of the pupil should ensue. Following removal of the light source the pupil should return to its original size. The procedure should be repeated for the other eye. There should also be a consensual reaction to the light source, i.e. both eyes constrict when the light source is applied to the one. Non-reactive pupils can be caused by an expanding mass, e.g. a blood clot exerting pressure on the third cranial

nerve; a fixed and dilated pupil may be due to herniation of the medial temporal lobe (Bassett & Makin, 2000). The reaction should be documented as 'B' for brisk, 'N' for no reaction and sl or 'S' for some or sluggish reaction (follow local policy). Note that lens implants or cataracts may prevent the pupil from constricting to light (Waterhouse, 2005).

- *Equality*: both pupils should be the same shape, size and react equally to light.

The Glasgow Coma Scale

The GCS (see Figure 6.1) was originally developed to grade the severity and outcome of traumatic head injury (Teasdale & Jennett, 1974). It is simple to use, requires no special equipment and is a good predictor of outcome (Woodrow, 2000). It is now used worldwide to assess the level of consciousness (Mallett & Dougherty, 2000) allowing:

- *Standardisation* of the clinical observations of patients with impaired consciousness
- *Progress monitoring* of patients undergoing intracranial surgery with minimal variation and subjectivity in the clinical assessment
- An *indication* of prognosis.

(Shah, 1999)

The GCS assesses the two aspects of consciousness:

- *Arousal* or *wakefulness*: being aware of the environment
- *Awareness*: demonstrating an understanding of what the practitioner has said through an ability to perform tasks.

The 15-point scale assesses the patient's level of consciousness by evaluating three behavioural responses: eye opening, verbal response and motor response (Fairley, 2005 and Waterhouse, 2005). Each will now be discussed in turn.

Eye opening

Assessment of eye opening involves the evaluation of arousal, the first aspect of consciousness. If the patient's eyes are closed, their

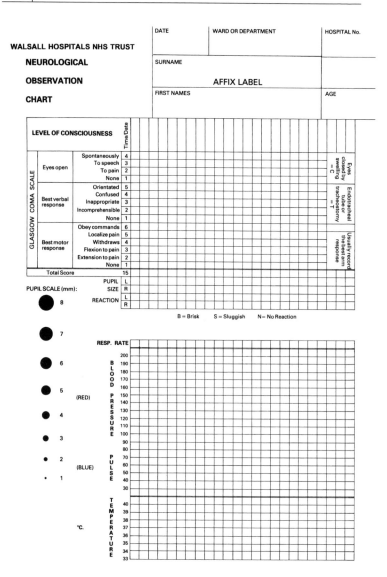

Fig 6.1 Neurological observation chart (Walsall Hospital NHS Trust)

state of arousal is assessed according to the degree of stimulation required to secure eye opening. Eye opening (arousal) is always the first measurement undertaken as part of the GCS, because without it cognition cannot occur (Aucken & Crawford, 1998). If the patient's eyes are swollen, opening them may not be possible (Mallett & Dougherty, 2000). The scoring is as follows.

- *Score 4 – spontaneously*: eyes open without the need for speech or touch (Fairley, 2005); optimum response.
- *Score 3 – to speech*: eyes open in response to a verbal stimulus (usually the patient's name) without touching the patient (Waterhouse, 2005). Begin at normal volume and raise your voice if necessary (Woodrow, 2005) using clear commands (Fairley, 2005).
- *Score 2 – to pain*: eyes open in response to central pain only, e.g. trapezium squeeze, suborbital pressure, pressure in the jaw margin. Note that painful stimuli should be employed only if the patient fails to respond to firm and clear commands (Mallett & Dougherty, 2000).
- *Score 1 – no response*: no eye opening despite verbal and central pain stimulus.

Record 'C' if the patient is unable to open the eyes due to swelling, ptosis or a dressing.

Verbal response

Assessment of verbal response involves the evaluation of awareness, the second aspect of consciousness. Comprehension of what the practitioner has said and functioning areas of the higher centres and ability to articulate and express a reply are being evaluated (Waterhouse, 2005). Dysphasia or inability to speak can be caused by any damage to the speech centres in the brain, e.g. following intracranial surgery or head injury.

It is important to ascertain the patient's acuity of hearing and understanding of language prior to assessing this response (Adam & Osborne, 1999). The lack of speech may not always indicate a falling level of consciousness (Mallett & Dougherty, 2000). In addition, some patients may require a lot of stimulation to maintain their concentration while answering questions. The amount of stimulation required should be documented as part of baseline assessment (Aucken & Crawford, 1998). The scoring is as follows:

- *Score 5 – orientated*: the patient can tell the practitioner who they are, where they are and the day, the current year and month (avoid using the day of the week or date) (Woodrow, 2005).
- *Score 4 – confused*: the patient can hold a conversation with the practitioner, but cannot answer the preceding questions accurately (Fairley, 2005).
- *Score 3 – inappropriate words*: the patient tends to use single words more than sentences and conversational exchange is absent (Fairley, 2005).
- *Score 2 – incomprehensible sounds*: the patient's response is made up of incomprehensible sounds such as moans or groans (Mooney & Comerford, 2003) but no discernable words. A verbal stimulus together with a pain stimulus may be needed to get a response from the patient. This type of patient is not aware of their surroundings (Mooney & Comerford, 2003).
- *Score 1 – no response*: no response from the patient despite both verbal and physical stimuli (Fairley, 2005).

Record 'D' if the patient is dysphasic and 'T' if the patient has a tracheal or tracheostomy tube *in situ*.

Motor response

The motor response is designed to ascertain the patient's ability to obey a command and to localize, withdraw or assume abnormal body positions in response to a painful stimulus (Adam & Osborne, 2005). If the patient does not respond by obeying commands the response to a painful stimulus should then be assessed.

In the past the application of a peripheral painful stimulus (pressure applied to fingernail bed) has been advocated (Teasdale

& Jennett, 1974). However, this can be traumatic and is no longer recommended. In addition, a peripheral stimulus may only elicit a spinal reflex, which does not involve cerebral function (Shah, 1999). It can cause patients to pull their fingers away from the source of pain; only a central painful stimulus will demonstrate localization to pain (Waterhouse, 2005).

A true localizing response involves the patient bringing an arm up to chin level, to pull an oxygen mask off, for example (Waterhouse, 2005). To elicit this response, the trapezium squeeze, supraorbital ridge pressure or pressure on the jaw margin are recommended. To avoid soft tissue injury no stimulus should be applied for more than 10 s (Waterhouse, 2005). In addition, when applying a stimulus it is best practice to start off with light pressure and increase to elicit a response (Sheppard & Wright, 2000).

- *Score 6 – obeys commands*: ask the patient to stick his tongue out; never ask a patient just to squeeze your hand, as this could elicit a primitive grasp response; ensure you ask them to let go. As it is important to establish that the response is not just a reflex movement, it is important to ask the patient to carry out two different commands (Bassett & Makin, 2000).
- *Score 5 – localizes to central pain, if the patient does not respond to verbal stimuli*: the patient purposely moves an arm in an attempt to remove the cause of the pain. Supraorbital ridge pressure is considered to be the most reliable technique, as this is less likely to be misinterpreted (Fairley, 2005).
- *Score 4 – withdrawing from pain*: the patient flexes or bends arm towards the source of the pain, but fails to locate the source of the pain (Waterhouse, 2005). There is no wrist rotation.
- *Score 3 – flexion to pain*: the patient flexes or bends the arm. It is characterized by internal rotation and adduction of the shoulder and flexion of the elbow, and is much slower than normal flexion (Fairley, 2005).

- *Score 2 – extension to pain*: the patient extends the arm by straightening the elbow, sometimes associated with internal shoulder and wrist rotation, sometimes referred to as decerebrate posture (Waterhouse, 2005).
- *Score 1 – no response*: no response to central painful stimuli.

Within each category each level of response is allocated a numerical value, on a scale of increasing neurological deterioration (Waterhouse, 2005). By assigning a numerical value to the level of response to the individual criteria in each section, three figures are obtained which add up to a maximum score of 15 and a minimum of 3. Coma is said to exist when GCS is 8 (Ibarran & Price, 1998). A total score of 12 or less should give rise to concern (Woodrow, 2000). A reduction in motor score by 1 or an overall deterioration of 2 is significant and should be reported (Cree, 2003, NICE, 2003 and Smith, 2003). Although aggregate scores are often documented, the weighting of scores between eye, verbal and motor responses remains untested (Woodrow, 2000). Therefore, documenting responses individually may provide a clearer indication of remaining functions and deficits (Waterhouse, 2005). The neurological observation chart depicted in Figure 6.1 incorporates the GCS.

The frequency of GCS monitoring should be individualized to the patient's needs (Woodrow, 2000). Instead of stressing the numerical score attached to each response, it is far better to define the responses in descriptive terms.

There are difficulties with using the GCS on an ICU, particularly in sedated, ventilated, head-injured patients. The GCS is designed to assess cerebral function, not sedation scores (Cree, 2003). Differences in scores of 2 or more have been reported on the same patients by different practitioners (Holdgate, 2006), which reiterates the recommendation that clinical decisions should not be based solely upon GCS (Holdgate, 2006), but be used as a component of monitoring neurological function. GCS should only be used as an aid to patient assessment (Adam & Osborne, 2005).

TREATMENT OF A PATIENT WITH ALTERED CONSCIOUSNESS LEVEL

Review ABC

- Review airway, breathing and circulation (Wyatt *et al.*, 2006). A compromised airway, inadequate breathing or inadequate circulation can lead to altered consciousness level. In addition, these can predispose to the development of cerebral oedema; this causes an increase in intracranial pressure, which can exacerbate an existing cerebral injury (Smith, 2003). Exclude or treat hypoxia, hypercapnia and hypotension (Resuscitation Council UK, 2006).
- Assess the need for an oropharyngeal or nasopharyngeal airway (see pages 26–9). It may be necessary to request expert help – tracheal intubation could be required.
- Administer high concentration of oxygen.

Assess consciousness level

- Initially assess the patient's consciousness level using the simple AVPU scale (see page 111). Record the GCS in the later full patient assessment to provide a more specific measurement of consciousness level (Smith, 2003). The GCS should all be recorded in patients with a head injury (NICE, 2003).
- Examine the pupils (size, equality and reaction to light).

Exclude hypoglycaemia

- Perform bedside blood glucose measurement (Figure 6.2). Hypoglycaemia is a deficiency of glucose in the circulation, causing muscular weakness, impaired consciousness level and sweating (McFerran & Martin, 2003). Potentially fatal, it causes 2.4% of deaths in diabetic patients on insulin; even mild episodes can lead to cerebral damage (Wyatt *et al.*, 2006). As hypoglycaemia can mimic any neurological presentation, always exclude it in any patient with altered consciousness level

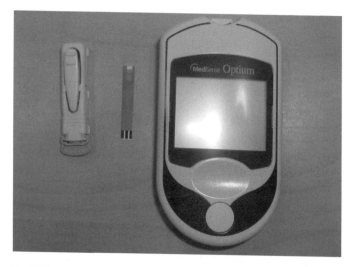

Fig 6.2 Bedside assessment of blood sugar

(Wyatt *et al.*, 2006). Normal blood glucose is 3.5–5.8 mmol/l: cognitive function deteriorates at < 3 mmol/l and symptoms usually only present if < 2.5 mmol/l (Wyatt *et al.*, 2006).

- If the blood glucose is < 3 mmol/l, administer 25–50 ml of 50% dextrose i.v. (Smith, 2003). Draw up the dextrose using a quill (because of its viscosity) and, because 50% dextrose is hypertonic and can cause thrombophlebitis, always administer a normal saline flush following injection (Wyatt *et al.*, 2006). If securing i.v. access is difficult, glucagon 1 mg i.m. can be administered. In some patients it may be appropriate to administer a fast-acting carbohydrate, e.g. Lucozade, sugar lumps, Dextrosol, followed by milk and biscuits (Wyatt *et al.*, 2006).

Place the patient horizontal in a lateral recovery position

- Place the patient in a lateral recovery position (Figure 6.3). In altered consciousness level, the airway is at risk. Regurgitated gastric contents, debris in the mouth or upper airway, loose

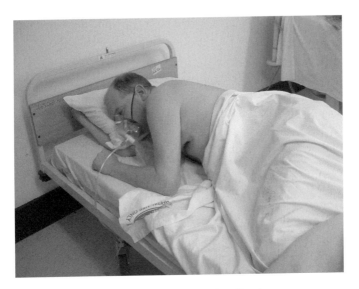

Fig 6.3 The recovery position (usually modified using pillows)

dentures or mechanical obstruction arising from structures in the mouth, e.g. the tongue and epiglottis, can all compromise the airway (Quinn, 1998). The recommended procedure for placing the patient in the recovery position is described on pages 32–3. In hospital, this procedure is often modified, e.g. using pillows.

Exclude reversible drug-induced causes

- Check the patient's drug chart for reversible drug-induced causes of altered consciousness level; administer the appropriate antagonist, where available, e.g. naloxone for opioid toxicity (Resuscitation Council UK, 2006).

CONCLUSION

Altered consciousness level is a common finding in the critically ill patient. Potentially life threatening, the initial priorities are to ensure a clear airway, adequate breathing and adequate circulation. Identifying and, where possible, treating the underlying cause is important.

REFERENCES

Adam, S, & Osborne, S. (2005) *Critical Care Nursing Science and Practice,* 2nd edn. Oxford University Press, Oxford.

American Heart Association (2005) 2005 American Heart Association Guidelines for cardiopulmonary resuscitation and emergency cardiovascular care. *Circulation* **112,** 24 (Suppl.).

Bassett, C. & Makin, L., eds (2000) *Caring for the Seriously Ill Patient.* Arnold, London.

Bersten, AD, Soni, N, Oh, TE. (2003) *Oh's Intensive Care Manual,* 5th edn. Butterworth-Heinemann, London, UK.

Bingham, E. (2004) Epilepsy: diagnosis and support for people with epilepsy. *Practice Nursing* **15,** 64–70.

Cree, C. (2003) Acquired brain injury: acute management. *Nursing Standard* **18,** 45–54.

Dean, R. (2005) Emergency first aid for nurses. *Nursing Standard* **20,** 57–65.

Diebel, G. (1999) The management of hypoglycaemia in type1 and type 2 diabetes. *Br J Community Nursing* **4,** 454–460.

Eastwick-Field, P. (1996) Resuscitation: basic life support. *Nursing Standard* **10,** 49–56.

Fairley, D. (2005) Using a coma scale to assess patient consciousness levels. *Nursing Times* **101,** 38–47.

Fulstow, R, & Smith, G. (1993) The new recovery position, a cautionary tale. *Resuscitation* **26,** 89–91.

Geraghty, M. (2005) Nursing the unconscious patient. *Nursing Standard* **20,** 54–64.

Handley, A. (1993) Recovery position. *Resuscitation* **26,** 93–95.

Hayes, C. (2004) Clinical skills: practical guide for managing adults with epilepsy. *Br J Nursing* **13,** 380–387.

Holdgate, A. (2006) Variability in agreement between physicians and nurses when measuring the Glasgow Coma Scale in the emergency department limits its clinical usefulness. *Emergency Medicine Australasia* **18,** 379–384.

McFerran, T, & Martin, E. (2003) *Minidictionary for Nurses*. Oxford University Press, Oxford.

Mallett, J. & Dougherty, L. (2000), eds. *The Royal Marsden Hospital Manual of Clinical Nursing Procedures*. Blackwell Science, Oxford.

Mooney, GP, & Comerford, DM. (2003) Neurological observations. *Nursing Times* **99,** 24–25.

National Institute for Clinical Excellence (2003) *Head Injury, Triage, Assessment, Investigation and Early Management of Head Injury in Infants, Children and Adults*. NICE, London.

Quinn, T. (1998) Cardiopulmonary resuscitation: new European guidelines. *Br J Nursing* **7,** 1070–1077.

Rathgeber, J, Panzer, W, Gunther, U *et al.* (1996) Influence of different types of recovery positions on perfusion indices of the forearm. *Resuscitation* **32,** 13–17.

Resuscitation Council (UK) (2005) *Guidelines 2005*. Resuscitation Council (UK), London.

Resuscitation Council (UK) (2006) *Advanced Life Support,* 5th edn. Resuscitation Council (UK), London.

Ryan, A, Larsen, P, Galletly, D. (2003) Comparison of heart rate variability in supine, and left and right lateral positions. *Anaesthesia* **58,** 432–436.

Shah, S. (1999) Neurological assessment. *Nursing Standard* **13,** 49–54.

Smith, G. (2003) *ALERT Acute Life-Threatening Events Recognition and Treatment,* 2nd edn. University of Portsmouth, Portsmouth.

Teasdale, G. & Jennett, B. (1974) Assessment of coma and impaired consciousness: a practical scale. *Lancet* **2,** 81–84.

Turner, S, Turner, I, Chapman, D *et al.* (1997) A comparative study of the 1992 and 1997 recovery positions for use in the UK. *Resuscitation* **39,** 153–160.

Waterhouse, C. (2005) The Glasgow Coma Scale and other neurological observations. *Nursing Standard* **19,** 56–64.

Wyatt, J, Illingworth, R, Graham, C *et al.* (2006) *Oxford Handbook of Emergency Medicine,* 3rd edn. Oxford University Press, Oxford.

7 | Treating a Patient with Oliguria

INTRODUCTION

Monitoring urine output is a very useful guide to the adequacy of cardiac output, splanchnic perfusion and renal function (Andrews & Nolan, 2005). The presence of oliguria is an early sign that the patient's general condition could be deteriorating. It is usually related to hypovolaemia caused by restricted fluid intake or excessive fluid loss (Docherty & Coote, 2006). Early recognition of oliguria and renal dysfunction allows the commencement of measures to reverse ischaemia/toxicity and to re-establish urine output and renal function (Leach, 2004).

Identifying the cause of the oliguria and managing it appropriately are essential: failure to instigate the necessary treatment promptly could result in further deterioration of the patient and progression to acute renal failure (Ahern & Philpot, 2002), a life-threatening condition that is becoming increasingly common in critically ill patients (Hilton, 2006 and Gwinnutt, 2006).

The aim of this chapter is to understand the treatment of a patient with oliguria.

LEARNING OBJECTIVES

At the end of this chapter the reader will be able to:

❏ Discuss the importance of fluid balance
❏ Outline normal and abnormal urine output
❏ List the causes of oliguria
❏ Discuss the signs of hypovolaemia
❏ Describe the signs of oliguria
❏ Describe the recognition of retention of urine

❏ Discuss the importance of fluid therapy in oliguria
❏ Outline the treatment for oliguria.

IMPORTANCE OF FLUID BALANCE

Role of fluid balance

Fluid balance is essential for the normal functioning of all the systems in the body: it maintains body temperature and cell shape, and is necessary for the transportation of nutrients, gases and waste products (Tortora & Grabowski, 2002 and Docherty & Coote, 2006).

Fluids can be intracellular or extracellular and can be divided into three categories:

- *Isotonic*: i.e. a fluid that has the same osmotic pressure as another fluid
- *Hypotonic*: i.e. a fluid that has a lower osmotic pressure than another fluid
- *Hypertonic*: i.e. a fluid that has a greater osmotic pressure than another fluid.
  (Docherty & Coote, 2006 and McFerran & Martin, 2003)

Regulation of fluid balance

Fluid balance is regulated by several complex regulators:

- *Kidneys*: if 2% of body fluid is lost, the kidneys will re-absorb more water from the filtrate (resulting in concentrated urine), i.e. the presence of dark, concentrated urine indicates renal compensation for a deranged fluid balance
- *Anti-diuretic hormone (ADH)*: released from the posterior pituitary gland as a response to decreased circulatory blood volume and increased serum osmolarity, ADH increases the re-absorption of water
- *Renin and angiotensin response*: if blood flow to the kidneys diminishes, renin is released which, after being converted to angiotensin II, is a powerful vasoconstrictor (i.e. it increases blood pressure)

- *Aldosterone*: secreted by the adrenal cortex, aldosterone helps to regulate the re-absorption of sodium and water.

(Source: Docherty & Coote, 2006)

Monitoring fluid balance

Monitoring fluid balance in the critically ill patient is paramount. Numerous factors can affect fluid status, including physiological mechanisms, disease processes and treatment side-effects (Sheppard, 2000). Fluid input and output should be closely monitored at least hourly and the following should be recorded:

- Oral intake
- Urine output
- Wound and nasogastric drainage
- All drug and fluid infusions.

(Adam & Osborne, 2005)

Monitoring the patient for signs of fluid loss/gain should also be undertaken (Table 7.1). It is important to be aware of the patient's fluid status and current fluid therapies and anticipate urine and electrolyte abnormalities output. Careful monitoring of the fluid balance chart must be maintained and this should include all input and output.

Daily measurement of serum sodium, potassium, urea and creatinine together with 24-h urine volume are required to assess fluid and electrolyte balance. Monitoring the patient's weight on a daily basis can be helpful. In addition, fluid balance charts from the preceding few days should be compared with serum and urine urea and electrolyte values. This will help evaluate the patient's response to fluid administration and will guide the fluid regime over the next 12–24h (Gosling, 1999).

Fluid balance should be regularly reviewed in combination with respiratory and haemodynamic measurements, e.g. respiratory rate, blood pressure and central venous pressure. Fluid and electrolyte overload is sometimes difficult to avoid and is commonly found in patients with multiorgan failure (Gosling, 1999).

Table 7.1 Systemic signs of fluid loss and fluid gain (Source: Sheppard & Wright, 2000)

System	Signs in fluid loss	Signs in fluid gain
Respiratory	Respiratory rate ↑	Orthopnoea Pulmonary oedema
Cardiovascular	Heart rate ↑ Low volume pulse Blood pressure ↓ Central venous pressure ↓	Heart rate ↑ Blood pressure ↑ Central venous pressure ↑ Distension of neck veins
Renal	Urine output ↓ (or ↑ in diabetes insipidus)	Urine output ↑ or ↓ depending on underlying cause and renal function
Skin	Dry	Pitting oedema may be present

NORMAL AND ABNORMAL URINE OUTPUT

Composition of urine and specific gravity

Urine is composed of 95% water and 5% solutes, e.g. urea, creatinine, sodium (Richardson, 2006b). It is slightly acidic (pH 6.0) and has a specific gravity of 1.010–1.030 (specific gravity of water is 1.000) (Wilson, 2005). The specific gravity of urine is a measure of urine osmolality (Redmond *et al.*, 2004), the normal range being 1.001–1.035. Urine of high specific gravity is concentrated and urine with a low specific gravity is dilute (Terrill, 2002). High values are indicative of dehydration and low values are found with high fluid intake, diabetes insipidus, renal failure, hypercalcaemia or hypokalaemia (Wilson, 2005).

Urine output

Filtration, selective reabsorption and tubular secretion are the three processes involved in urine output (Waugh & Grant, 2006 and Richardson, 2006a). The average urine output in a healthy adult is 1500–2000 ml/day (Smith, 2003).

The presence of urine does not necessarily mean that renal function is adequate: although the patient may be producing adequate volumes of urine, the ability of the kidneys to reabsorb water and electrolytes may be disrupted, hence the importance of monitoring serum and urinary urea, creatine and electrolytes (Ahern & Philpot, 2002).

Prerequisites for normal urine output

Prerequisites for normal urine output include:

- *Adequate renal perfusion*: renal blood flow is approximately 1200 ml/min (Richardson, 2006). This remains constant if the mean blood pressure is between 70 and 170 mmHg (Smith, 2003). It is kept constant by
- *Normal renal function*
- *No obstruction to the flow of urine*: if the patient has a urinary catheter, the patency and correct positioning should be checked.

Definitions of abnormal urine output

Listed below are the generally accepted definitions of abnormal urine output:

- *Oliguria*: 100–400 ml in 24 h
- *Anuria*: <100 ml in 24 h
- *Absolute anuria*: 0 ml in 24 h.

(Smith, 2003 and Docherty & Coote, 2006)

CAUSES OF OLIGURIA

In the critically ill patient the most common cause of oliguria is renal perfusion or pre-renal impairment caused by hypovolaemia (Ahern & Philpot, 2002). Absolute anuria is quite rare and is most likely to be associated with a blocked catheter (Ahern & Philpot, 2002 and Adam & Osborne, 2005). Retention of urine should always be excluded as a possible cause of poor urine output.

RECOGNITION OF RETENTION OF URINE

In all patients with oliguria, it is important to exclude retention of urine. Retention of urine can be caused by the effects of opioid analgesia on the bladder sphincter control, removing the sensation of a full bladder (more common in men, especially if there are existing symptoms of prostatism) (Gwinnutt, 2006).

A reasonably full bladder can hold approximately 500 ml of urine, although it can expand to hold more than 1 l if necessary (Richardson, 2006b). If the bladder is full it can be palpated above the symphisis pubis (Marieb, 2006). An empty bladder is impalpable (Talley & O'Connor, 2001). To check for a distended bladder:

- Palpate the abdomen above the pubic symphysis (Figure 7.1). If the bladder is distended the swelling is usually regular, smooth, firm and oval-shaped; it can occasionally reach as high as the umbilicus (Talley & O'Connor, 2001).
- Percuss the abdomen above the pubic symphosis. Following the general principle of percussing from resonance to dullness,

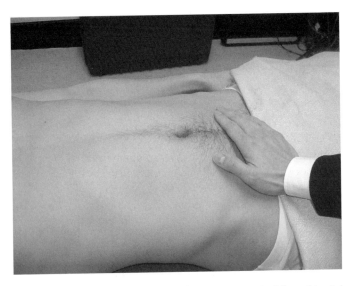

Fig 7.1 Palpate the abdomen above the pubic symphysis to check for a distended bladder

percuss from the level of the umbilicus, parallel to the pubis, and progress down the mid-line towards the pubic bone (Epstein *et al.*, 2003). The supra-pubic region is usually tympanic (Epstein *et al.*, 2003) and a dull sound on percussion over this area may indicate a distended bladder (Talley & O'Connor, 2001 and Epstein *et al.*, 2003).

SIGNS OF HYPOVOLAEMIA

In the critically ill patient, oliguria is usually related to hypovolaemia, caused by restricted fluid intake or excessive fluid loss (Ahern & Philpott, 2002). Causes of excessive fluid loss include haemorrhage, burns, diarrhoea, vomiting, sweating and diuretic therapy (Macklin *et al.*, 2002). Early signs of hypovolaemia include:

- Thirst
- Dry lips
- Dry oral mucosa
- Concentrated urine
- Reduced urine output
- Mild tachycardia.

(Mehta *et al.*, 2002)

Late signs of hypovolaemia include:

- Tachycardia
- Hypotension
- Altered level of consciousness, e.g. agitation, confusion and unconsciousness
- Oliguria
- Prolonged capillary refill time.

(Mehta *et al.*, 2002)

IMPORTANCE OF FLUID THERAPY IN OLIGURIA

Oliguria which has been caused by a fall in blood pressure, renal blood flow or cardiac output is potentially reversible if appropriate fluid therapy is immediately administered (Smith, 2003). Fluid therapy (fluid challenge), a key treatment strategy in the resuscitation of the critically ill patient (Docherty & Coote, 2006), is the only treatment that has been shown to be effective in preventing acute renal failure in the general ward setting (Mehta *et al.*, 2002). The aim is to produce a significant and rapid increase in plasma volume (Singer & Webb, 2005). This initial treatment will hopefully stabilize the patient's condition, thus buying time so that expert help can be sought and a more definite diagnosis made (Gwinnutt, 2006).

The fluid therapy of choice is usually an isotonic crystalloid (e.g. 0.9% normal saline, Hartmann's solution or Ringers' lactate), unless the patient also requires replacement of blood components such as red blood cells (Doherty & Coote, 2006). Fluids containing dextrose are not used for initial resuscitation because they rapidly distribute throughout both the intracellular and extracellular fluid compartments in the body, with very little remaining in the circulation (Gwinnutt, 2006).

A bolus of fluid, usually 500 ml of a crystalloid, is administered over approximately 15 min and then the patient is observed for signs of improvement, e.g. decreased respiratory and pulse rates, a rise in blood pressure and improved level of consciousness (Gwinnutt, 2006). The fluid bolus should be repeated until the blood pressure, central venous pressure (CVP) and urine output are satisfactory (Adam & Osborne, 2005).

It is important to consider cardiac and renal function when attempting to administer large volumes of fluid (Doherty & Coote, 2006). However, even patients with cardiogenic shock should receive a fluid challenge, e.g. 250 ml of crystalloid (Smith, 2003).

TREATMENT OF A PATIENT WITH OLIGURIA

The primary objective of treating a patient with oliguria is to identify the cause so that the most appropriate treatment can be instigated. The most common cause of oliguria in the critically ill patient is reduced renal perfusion or pre-renal impairment due to hypovolaemia, which should be suspected first; absolute anuria due to obstruction is very rare and is probably due to a blocked catheter (Ahern & Philpot, 2002).

If the patient has oliguria:

- Check for obstruction to urine flow: exclude distended bladder and retention of urine. The abdomen should be examined in order to establish if the bladder is distended (Smith, 2003) (see above). If the bladder is palpable, and the patient is unable to urinate, insert a urinary catheter (Box 7.1). In addition, in men a rectal examination will also need to be undertaken because an enlarged prostate could be the cause (Smith, 2003).
- Exclude the possibility of a blocked urinary catheter (Adam & Osborne, 2005). The catheter should be carefully checked to ensure that it is not blocked and is functioning correctly (particularly if absolute anuria is present):
  - check that the catheter and the catheter drainage tubing are not kinked: inspect the system and remove any kinks;
  - check that the catheter and the catheter drainage tubing are still connected and not leaking;
  - check that the catheter and the catheter drainage tubing are not blocked, e.g. by blood clots. If a blocked catheter is suspected and a three-way catheter is in place, irrigate it;
  - gently flush the catheter with sterile water, checking that the same volume of water returns (Ahern & Philpot, 2002).
- Check that the catheter has not become dislodged or was not incorrectly placed: a new catheter may need to be inserted (Ahern & Philpot, 2002). Perform bladder washout if there is a lot of debris in the urine or if blood clots are present.
- Perform urinalysis. If there is inadequate renal perfusion, any urine formed will have a low sodium content and a high osmolality (Smith, 2003). The urine will be concentrated and the specific gravity will be high.
- If the patient does not have a urinary catheter *in situ*, insert one (Smith, 2003). Suggested procedures for male and female catheterization are detailed in Box 7.1.

Box 7.1 Suggested procedures for male and female urinary catheterization

A suggested procedure for male catheterization:

- Explain the procedure to the patient.
- Assemble the necessary equipment.
- Wash hands and ensure the patient has privacy.
- Place an incontinence pad or similar underneath the patient's buttocks.
- Using an aseptic technique, open the catheterization pack etc. onto the top of the trolley.
- Don sterile gloves.
- Position the sterile towel over the patients exposed groin
- Gently grasp the penis laterally behind the glans using a sterile swab.
- Carefully bring the penis through the opening of the sterile towel.
- Select an appropriate catheter following local protocols. A balloon (Foley) two-way catheter, i.e. one for urine drainage and the other for balloon inflation, is commonly used (Dougherty & Lister, 2004). Select the smallest gauge catheter possible. This will usually be a size 12 (Dougherty & Lister, 2004).
- While gently retracting the foreskin (if present), cleanse the shaft, glans and urethral meatus using soap and water, taking care to swab in a direction away from the urethral orifice.
- Slowly instill the antiseptic gel (2% lignocaine gel) into the urethra. Massage it along the urethra and then wait 5 min for it to take effect (British Association of Urology Nurses, 1998–9).
- While holding the penis at right angles to the pelvis, gently insert the catheter approximately 15–25 cm until a flow of urine is noted. Then insert it a further 1–2 cm and inflate the balloon with sterile water.
- Observe the patient for signs of pain, discomfort and bleeding from the urethra; gently withdraw the catheter slightly until resistance can be felt.

Continued

- Connect the catheter to a urine drainage bag; one with an hourly urine measurement facility may be required if close monitoring of urine output is required (see Figure 7.2). Ensure the bag is secured to the bed and not touching the floor.
- Gently re-position the foreskin (if present) and ensure the patient is comfortable.
- Record the amount, colour and consistency of residual urine.
- Document the procedure in the patient's notes.
- Monitor urine output.

(Sources: Dougherty & Lister, 2004)

A suggested procedure for female catheterization:

- Explain the procedure to the patient.
- Assemble the necessary equipment.
- Ensure the patient has privacy.
- Help the patient to adopt a supine position, with knees bent, hips flexed and feet resting approximately 60 cm apart.
- Ensure adequate lighting.
- Wash and dry hands.
- Expose the patient's groin and place an incontinence pad or similar underneath the patient's buttocks.
- Using an aseptic technique, open the catheterization pack etc. onto the top of the trolley.
- Don sterile gloves.
- Position sterile towels over the patient's thighs.
- Using a sterile swab, gently separate the labia minora to expose the urethral meatus.
- Gently clean the urethral orifice with either 0.9% sodium chloride or an antiseptic solution, using single downward strokes.
- Slowly instil the antiseptic gel (2% lignocaine gel) into the urethra.
- Insert the catheter into the urethral orifice in an upward and backward direction, advancing it 5–6 cm.
- Inflate the balloon with sterile water following the manufacturer's recommendations.

- Observe the patient for signs of pain, discomfort and bleeding from the urethra; gently withdraw the catheter slightly until resistance can be felt.
- Connect the catheter to a urine drainage bag; one with an hourly urine measurement facility may be required if close monitoring of urine output is required (see Figure 7.2). Ensure the bag is secured to the bed and not touching the floor.
- Assist the patient into a comfortable position.
- Record the amount, colour and consistency of residual urine.
- Document the procedure in the patient's notes.
- Monitor urine output.

- Administer a bolus of fluid (usually 500 ml of a crystalloid) over approximately 15 min and then observe the patient for signs of improvement, e.g. decreased respiratory and pulse rates, a rise in blood pressure and improved level of consciousness (Gwinnutt, 2006). Repeat the fluid bolus until the blood pressure, CVP and urine output are satisfactory (Adam & Osborne, 2005). If the patient has cardiogenic shock, administer smaller volumes of fluid, e.g. 250 ml of crystalloid (Smith, 2003).
- Review the use of nephrotoxic drugs. Carefully review the patient's drug chart to check whether nephrotoxic drugs are being administered: a senior clinician will probably decide to stop these drugs (Smith, 2003). Nephrotoxic drugs include non-steroidal anti-inflammatory drugs (NSAIDs), frusemide, gentamicin and cyclosporin (Leach, 2004). The nephrotoxic effects of these drugs can be exacerbated by hypovolaemia (Ahern & Philpot, 2002). NSAIDs, e.g. aspirin, ibuprofen and naproxin, antibiotics, a group of drugs commonly used for pain relief in rheumatoid arthritis, act by inhibiting normal prostaglandin-induced vasodilation, resulting in renal arteriolar vasoconstriction (Leach, 2004).

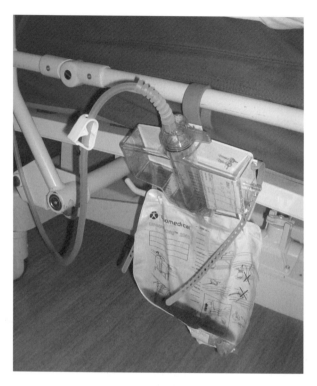

Fig 7.2 Hourly urine drainage bag

- Withhold diuretic therapy, unless clinical features confirm that there is fluid overload, e.g. oedema (Smith, 2003). Administering drugs, e.g. furosemide and dopamine, just to increase urine flow, without identifying and treating the underlying cause of the oliguria, will only delay correct diagnosis and treatment (Smith, 2003). Furosemide has been shown to be ineffective in preventing and treating acute renal failure (Hilton, 2006).
- Check the patient's blood chemistry:
  - *serum electrolytes*: in particular serum potassium as hyperkalaemia can be life threatening; normal range for potassium is 3.6–5 mmol (Marshall, 2002);

- *plasma urea*: normal range is 3.3–6.7 mmol; a raised urea is a feature of renal impairment (Marshall, 2002);
- *plasma creatinine*: the most reliable simple biochemical test of renal function; normal range is 60–120 mmol; a raised creatinine is a feature of renal impairment (Marshall, 2002).
- Check the acid base status by sending an arterial blood sample.
- Closely monitor fluid balance.

CONCLUSION

The presence of oliguria is an early sign that the patient's general condition could be deteriorating. It is usually related to hypovolaemia due to either restricted fluid intake or excessive fluid loss. Early recognition is paramount, so that the appropriate treatment, usually fluid resuscitation, can be promptly started. If oliguria is not effectively treated, acute renal failure can develop, which has high mortality rates.

REFERENCES

Adam, S, & Osborne, S. (2005) *Critical Care Nursing: Science and Practice*, 2nd edn. Oxford Medical Publications, Oxford.

Ahern, J, & Philpot, P. (2002) Assessing acutely ill patients on general wards. *Nursing Standard* **16,** 47–55.

Andrews, F, & Nolan, J. (2006) Critical care in the emergency department: monitoring the critically ill patient. *Emerg Med J* **23,** 561–564.

Docherty, B, & Coote, S. (2006) Fluid balance monitoring as part of track and trigger. *Nursing Times* **102,** 28–29.

Doherty, W. (2006) Male urine catheterization. *Nursing Standard* **20,** 57–64.

Hilton, R. (2006) Acute renal failure. *BMJ* **333** (7572), 786–790.

Gwinnutt, C. (2006) *Clinical Anaesthesia*, 2nd edn. Blackwell Publishing, Oxford.

Marshall, W. (2002) *Clinical Chemistry*, 4th edn. Mosby, London.

Mcferran, T, & Martin, E. (2003) *Minidictionary for Nurses.* Oxford University Press, Oxford.

Redmond, A, McDevitt, M, Barnes, S. (2004) Acute renal failure: recognition and treatment in ward patients. *Nursing Standard* **18,** 46–53.

Sheppard, M. (2000) Monitoring fluid balance in acutely ill patients. *Nursing Times* **96,** 39–40.

Talley, N, & O'Connor, S. (2001) *Clinical Examination: A Systematic Guide to Physical Diagnosis.* Blackwell Science, Oxford.

Terrill, B. (2002) *Renal Nursing – A Practical Approach.* Ausmed Publications, Victoria, Australia.

Tortora, GJ, & Grabowski, SR. (2003) *Principles of Anatomy and Physiology,* 10th edn. John Wiley & Sons Inc., NJ, USA.

Waugh, A, & Grant, A. (2006) *Ross and Wilson Anatomy and Physiology in Health and Illness,* 10th edn. Elsevier, Edinburgh.

Wilson, L. (2005) Urinalysis. *Nursing Standard* **19,** 51–54.

Woodrow, P. (2000) *Intensive Care Nursing: A Framework for Practice.* Routledge, London.

Treating a Patient with an Abnormal Temperature   **8**

INTRODUCTION

The body can only function effectively within a narrow temperature range (Trim, 2005). Any significant changes in temperature, either hypothermia or hyperpyrexia, can lead to life-threatening complications. Temperature monitoring in the acutely ill patient is therefore essential (Andrews & Nolan, 2006) and prompt detection and effective treatment of an abnormal temperature paramount.

The aim of this chapter is to understand how to treat a patient with an abnormal temperature.

LEARNING OBJECTIVES

At the end of this chapter the reader will be able to

❏ List the methods of monitoring the patient's temperature
❏ Define hypothermia
❏ List the risk factors for hypothermia
❏ Describe the effects of hypothermia
❏ Discuss the treatment of hypothermia
❏ Define pyrexia
❏ List the complications of hyperpyrexia
❏ Discuss the treatment of hyperpyrexia.

METHODS FOR MONITORING THE PATIENT'S TEMPERATURE

The patient's core temperature can be monitored at the tympanic membrane, oesophagus, bladder or rectum (Andrews & Nolan, 2006). An overview of the methods for monitoring temperature is provided below. A more comprehensive description can be found in Jevon & Ewens (2007).

Tympanic membrane

The tympanic membrane method for monitoring temperature is commonly used in the acutely ill patient. However, although practical and easy to do, poor technique can lead to inaccurate measurements. Correct technique following the manufacturer's recommendations is essential.

Oesophagus

The oesophagus method for monitoring temperature, using an oesophageal probe, is considered to be very reliable, but is suitable only for a patient who is intubated and sedated (Andrews & Nolan, 2006).

Bladder

The bladder method for monitoring temperature, using a bladder probe, is also considered to be very reliable, but is suitable only for a patient who is catheterized (Andrews & Nolan, 2006).

Rectum

The rectum method for monitoring temperature is now rarely used. Although rectal temperature is closest to core temperature (Schmitz *et al.*, 1994), it is unreliable in the critically ill patient because hypotension and gut ischaemia reduce the blood supply to the rectum (Holtzclaw, 1992) and the measurement is influenced by the contents in the rectum. The oesophagus and bladder methods are therefore considered superior to the rectum method (Andrews & Nolan, 2006).

DEFINITION OF HYPOTHERMIA

Hypothermia can be defined as < 35 °C (Petrone *et al.*, 2003).

It can be classified according to its severity:

- Mild hypothermia: 32–35 °C
- Moderate hypothermia: 30–32 °C
- Severe hypothermia: < 30 °C.

(Resuscitation Council UK, 2006)

Even mild hypothermia should be considered a medical emergency because of the rapid failure of thermoregulation and incremental decline of neuropsychological awareness (Nixdorf-Miller *et al.*, 2006).

RISK FACTORS FOR HYPOTHERMIA

Risk factors for hypothermia include:

- Poor accommodation
- Malnourishment
- Exposure to a cold environment
- Burns
- Coma and immobility
- Underlying illness, e.g. hypothyroidism
- Prescribed medications, e.g. antidepressants, barbiturates, opioids and benzodiazepines: they can adversely affect the body's ability to sense cold
- Alcohol: it prompts rapid cooling by effecting continuous peripheral vasodilation and inhibiting heat production by shivering
- Surgery.

(Sources: Kelly *et al.*, 2001 and Nixdorf-Miller *et al.*, 2006)

The elderly are particularly at risk of hypothermia because of:

- Reduced heat production due to loss of physiological reserves in chronic disease
- Increased heat loss due to malnutrition and diminished subcutaneous muscle and fat
- Impaired thermoregulation mainly because of primary or secondary pathologies of the central nervous system
- Inactivity.

(Beers *et al.*, 2000)

COMPLICATIONS OF HYPOTHERMIA

The complications of hypothermia can be classified according to its severity: mild, moderate or severe.

Mild hypothermia

- Confusion progressing to impaired judgement and apathy
- Inability to perform complex motor functions and ataxia
- 'Umbles': stumbles, mumbles, fumbles, and grumbles
- Vigorous shivering, tachycardia, tachypnoea, bronchospasm, peripheral vasoconstriction, increased cardiac output, hypertension
- Cold diuresis.

Moderate hypothermia

- Dazed consciousness, irrational behaviour, slurred speech, delirium, hallucinations
- Paradoxical undressing; hide and die
- Hyporeflexia; rigidity; shivering reduced
- Hypoventilation
- Progressive decrease in cardiac output and pulse; atrial and ventricular cardiac dysrhythmias.

Severe hypothermia

- Waves of shivering interspersed with lengthening dyspnoea followed by apnoea
- Decreased blood pressure, pulse and cardiac output; ventricular arrhythmias
- Coma.

(Nixdorf-Miller *et al.*, 2006)

TREATMENT OF A PATIENT WITH HYPOTHERMIA

Treatment of a patient with hypothermia will depend on its severity and the options available (Neno, 2005). Some guiding principles are to:

- If appropriate, remove or stop the cause of the hypo-thermia.
- Administer high concentrations of oxygen.
- Attach appropriate monitoring devices, e.g. pulse oximetry and ECG monitoring.
- Regularly assess the patient's vital signs: airway, breathing, circulation, consciousness level. In particular, closely monitor the patient during rewarming, because vasodilation and shivering increase cardiovascular instability and oxygen requirements are increased (Andrews & Nolan, 2006).
- Measure the patient's temperature every 30 min until the temperature is > 36 °C (Hodgetts *et al.*, 2004). Although, to avoid complications, rewarming should not usually exceed increases of 0.3–1.2 °C per hour, rapid re-warming of > 3 °C per hour may be necessary if there is severe hypothermia and cardiovascular instability (Carson, 1999).
- Provide passive external rewarming, e.g. reduce environmental factors (close windows etc.), remove any wet clothing or sheets, ensure the patient is lying on an insulated surface and apply blankets (Hodgetts *et al.*, 2004).
- If the patient's temperature < 34 °C, provide active external rewarming, e.g. warm air duvet, warmed (43 °C) i.v. fluids and humidified oxygen (42–46 °C) (Hodgetts *et al.*, 2004). For severe hypothermia, additional methods may be required, e.g. cardiopulmonary bypass (Resuscitation Council UK, 2006).
- Administer warmed i.v. fluids – large volumes may be required as the vascular space expands due to vasodilation during rewarming of the patient (Resuscitation Council UK, 2006).
- Closely monitor the patient for complications of hypothermia (see above) and report as appropriate.
- Ensure continuous ECG monitoring to detect cardiac arrhythmias and monitor urine output.
- Keep patient handling to a minimum, as it can precipitate cardiac arrhythmias.

Peripheral vasodilation may complicate active rewarming methods, resulting in a drop in core body temperature (Neno, 2005).

DEFINITION OF PYREXIA

Pyrexia can be defined as an abnormally high temperature. It can be graded as follows:

- *Low-grade pyrexia* (37–38 °C): causes include an inflammatory response due to mild infection, trauma, surgery, malignancy or thrombosis
- *Moderate to high-grade pyrexia* (38–40 °C): can be caused by a wound, urinary tract or respiratory infection
- *Hyperpyrexia* (>40 °C): causes include septicaemia, damage to the hypothalamus and environmental temperature.

(Source: Dougherty & Lister, 2005)

COMPLICATIONS OF HYPERPYREXIA

Complications of hyperpyrexia, which are dependent on its severity, can include:

- Tachycardia, ECG changes and cardiac failure
- Tachypnoea, increased oxygen consumption and respiratory alkalosis
- Confusion, delirium, convulsions and possibly coma
- Fluid loss and acute renal failure.

(Source: Jones *et al.*, 2003)

TREATMENT OF A PATIENT WITH HYPERPYREXIA

Hyperpyrexia can be life threatening. When treating hyperpyrexia:

- Remove the patient's clothing and ensure a cool environment.
- Provide active cooling, e.g. spray the patient's body with tepid tap water, use a fan, apply ice packs to the axilla, groin, neck and scalp (avoiding prolonged contact); aim for a cooling rate

of at least 0.1 °C/min (Wyatt *et al.*, 2006). Once the temperature is < 39 °C, stop active cooling because hypothermia may develop (Wyatt *et al.*, 2006).

- Do not administer antipyretics, e.g. aspirin or paracetamol (Wyatt *et al.*, 2006).
- Regularly assess the patient's vital signs.
- Monitor the patient's core body temperature.
- Monitor arterial blood gas analysis: particularly important if the patient has malignant hyperthermia as acidosis is common.
- Commence ECG monitoring to detect cardiac arrhythmias.
- Monitor fluid balance and administer fluids as prescribed (excessive sweating can lead to severe fluid loss).
- Monitor the patient's blood sugar as hypoglycaemia may develop – administer 50 ml 50% glucose if the blood sugar is < 3 mmol/l (Wyatt *et al.*, 2006).
- If possible, identify and treat the underlying cause.

CONCLUSION

The body can function effectively only within a narrow temperature range. Both hypothermia and hyperpyrexia can cause life-threatening complications. In this chapter the treatment for hypothermia and hyperpyrexia has been described.

REFERENCES

Andrews, F, & Nolan, J. (2006) Critical care in the emergency department: monitoring the critically ill patient. *Emerg Med J* **23**, 561–564.

Beers, M, & Berkow, R, eds. (2000) *The Merck Manual of Geriatrics,* 3rd edn. Merck & Co Inc.

Dougherty, L, & Lister, S, eds. (2005) *The Royal Marsden Hospital Manual of Clinical Nursing Procedures,* 6th edn. Blackwell Publishing, Oxford.

Jones, G, Endacott, R, Crouch, R. (2003) *Emergency Nursing Care.* Greenwich Medical Media Ltd, London.

Kelly, M, Ewens, B, Jevon, P. (2001) Hypothermia management. *Nursing Times* **97,** 36–37.

Neno, R. (2005) Hypothermia: assessment, treatment and prevention. *Nursing Standard* **19,** 47–55.

Nixdorf-Miller, A, Hunsaker, D, Hunsaker, J. (2006) Investigation of morbidity and mortality from exposure to environmental temperature extremes. *Arch Pathol Lab Med* **130,** 1297–1304.

Petrone, P, Kuncir, E, Asensio, J. (2003) Surgical management and strategies in the treatment of hypothermia and cold injury. *Emerg Med Clin North Am* **21,** 1165–1178.

Resuscitation Council UK (2006) *Advanced Life Support,* 5th edn. Resuscitation Council UK, London.

Trim, J. (2005) Monitoring temperature. *Nursing Times* **101,** 30–31.

Woodrow, P. (2000) *Intensive Care Nursing: A Framework for Practice.* Routledge, London.

Pain Management in the Critically Ill Patient

9

Tim Simmonds, BSc (Hons) RGN, PG Dip Pain Management, CPSN (ENB 100), CMS, OND, ENB 998. Independent and Supplementary Nurse Prescriber

INTRODUCTION

Pain often accompanies critical illness. Despite this, pain is often poorly managed even though it has been shown to be important in preventing adverse events and assisting the recovery process.

The aim of this chapter is help understand pain management in the critically ill patient.

LEARNING OBJECTIVES

At the end of this chapter the reader will be able to:

❏ Describe the physiology of pain
❏ List the effects of pain on the patient
❏ Discuss pain assessment
❏ List the routes of pain relief
❏ Discuss the use of analgesics
❏ Discuss non-pharmaceutical methods of pain relief
❏ List some problems associated with pain and analgesic drugs.

PHYSIOLOGY OF PAIN

The International Association for the Study of Pain describes pain as 'an unpleasant sensory and emotional experience associated with actual or potential tissue damage, or described in terms of such damage' (Merskey, 1979). It is a normal part of the body's defence mechanism, indicating that something is wrong.

Pain often accompanies critical illness; it is a symptom that can be invaluable in aiding diagnosis and may be thought of as the 'fifth vital sign' (JCAHO, 2001). Pain can result from disease, infection, trauma and from procedures undertaken on the patient: a plethora of clinical investigations and treatments existing today to aid diagnosis and treatment. Unfortunately, many of these have the penalty of also causing discomfort to the patient.

Pain is the result of complex neurochemical responses within the nervous system. In simple terms it can be described as a result of noxious stimuli of the peripheral nervous system causing sensory information to be passed via nerve fibres to the spinal cord. This is then passed via ascending fibres in the spinal cord to the thalamus and somatosensory cortex of the brain. This pain pathway can be affected by a variety of innate physiological and psychological mechanisms that exist to modulate the flow and perception of pain sensations to the brain. These include the release of the hormone-like substances endorphins, dynorphins and enkephalins and closure of the theoretical pain gate which lies with the dorsal horn of the spinal cord (Melzack and Wall, 1965). This gate can be closed by additional peripheral sensory input (the basis of transcutaneous electrostimulation) or by the influence of descending signals from the brain. Psychological factors also play an important part in the perception and subsequent reaction to pain (Turk, 1995) as well as response to treatment, the placebo response having a significant effect (Frank & Frank 1991). As a result, pain is a highly subjective and individual experience.

Pain may be classified as being either nociceptive or neuropathic (Box 9.1). Nociceptive pain results from stimulation of sensory receptors (nociceptors) as a result of excessive pressure, heat, cold or tissue injury. Neuropathic pain results from a lesion or dysfunction of the nervous system or pressure upon a nerve from another structure. As well as pain, alterations in sensation (either increased or decreased) and skin temperature changes can also occur. Postoperative pain is a typical form of nociceptive pain, sciatica being a form of neuropathic pain. Some patients, e.g. those with cancer, may experience a mixture of both forms.

Box 9.1 Simple pain descriptors

Nociceptive pain	*Neuropathic pain*
Sharp	Jumping
Aching	Shooting (like an electric shock)
Throbbing	Tingling (pins and needles)
Crushing (cardiac pain)	Hot/burning

EFFECTS OF PAIN ON THE PATIENT

Pain can lead to a variety of adverse physiological and psychological effects to the detriment of the patient:

- Increased anxiety and lack of sleep
- Delayed or reduced wound healing
- Atelectasis, hypoxaemia and hypercarbia
- Reduced cough and pneumonia
- Increased myocardial workload and oxygen consumption
- Delayed gastric emptying
- Increased cortisol secretion, decreased insulin secretion and hyperglycaemia.

(Smith, 2003)

In addition, it has been shown that inadequately treated acute pain can predispose a patient to develop chronic pain (Blyth *et al.*, 2003). It is therefore important that acute pain is treated not just on ethical grounds, but also to modify the response to injury (Cousins *et al.*, 2004).

PAIN ASSESSMENT

The initial assessment of a patient with pain should include a thorough assessment to:

- Identify the location, duration, frequency and intensity of the pain

- Identify the cause and nature of the pain
- Identify factors that relieve or exacerbate the pain, i.e. posture, movement, rest, massage, etc.
- Document previous and current analgesic use and its effectiveness
- Quantify the level and type of analgesia required according to the severity and type of pain being experienced
- Identify the presence of other pain problems, such as those related to a chronic condition, e.g. arthritis
- Provide a base line assessment in order to monitor the effectiveness of treatment
- Provide evidence of pain assessment for potential future medical legal issues, such as complaints and compensation claims against the hospital or a third party.

The management of pain during critical illness can be influenced by

- The patient's ability to take medication due to physical or cognitive difficulties
- Disordered physiology affecting the metabolism and excretion of drugs
- Communication problems such as language barrier, dysphagia, oral intubation and tracheostomy
- Psychological factors such as anxiety
- Previous analgesic use.

Pain assessment should be viewed as a continuous process, regular reassessment being associated with improved acute pain management (APM, 2005). Difficulties can arise when communication problems are encountered due to language barriers or dealing with the very young or cognitively impaired. The use of analgesia in the unconscious patient is difficult because of the problem of masking important neurological signs, particularly when using opiates due to their sedative effect.

Clues to the presence of pain in the elderly patient with dementia include verbal aggression, vocalizations such as moaning and shouting, body movements such as rocking and guarding, mood changes and general changes in behaviour. These and other indicators of pain have been incorporated into a variety of pain assessment tools, which can be applied to different clinical situations.

Physiological changes such as rise or fall in blood pressure and heart rate are unreliable, particularly in the critical care unit, if the patient is receiving drugs which affect the cardiovascular system such as inotropes and β-blockers (Arbor, 2000).

Psychological factors such as anxiety and depression can also effect pain perception and can have a major influence upon an individual's ability to cope with pain. Unfortunately, assessment of these influences can be time consuming and is rarely used in an acute situation (Hobbs & Hodgkinson, 2003).

Information concerning previous analgesia use is important. For example, patients may state they are allergic to a particular drug, but further questioning will reveal whether this is a true allergy or a known side-effect of the drug. It is also important to note any illicit drug-taking behaviour or use of drugs such as buphrenorphine and methadone as part of a substance abuse rehabilitation programme, as these can affect the choice, dose and tolerance of any subsequent analgesia.

A variety of pain assessment tools are available to enable repeated quantification of pain severity; nurses and patients prefer to use verbal rating scales (Briggs & Closs, 1999) (Figure 9.1). The concept of pain being the fifth vital sign, together with the high incidence of patients with pain in hospital, supports the inclusion of a pain score on the standard hospital observations chart (see Box 9.2). As with any other assessment tool, e.g. the critical care early warning score, it is of value only if it is consistently used, initiating appropriate and timely responses from staff should changes occur. The Leeds Assessment of Neuropathic Symptoms and Signs assessment tool has been developed to help diagnose neuropathic pain, which can present with different features from nociceptive pain (Bennet, 2001).

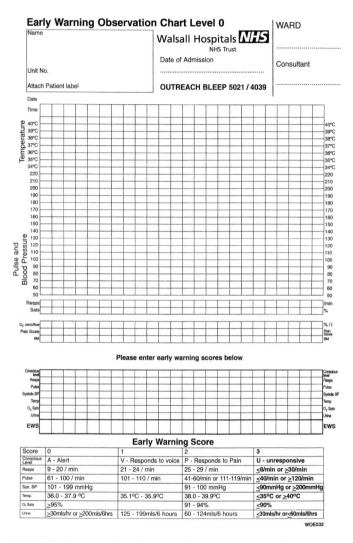

Fig 9.1 Standard ward observations chart incorporating early warning score and section for scoring pain (Walsall Hospital NHS Trust)

PRACTICAL CONSIDERATIONS

Not every patient will want or need a pharmacological response to a pain problem. Good nursing care, including correct positioning and attention to individual concerns, can do much to reduce anxiety and the impact of pain, improving the patient's ability to cope with its effects. This has in turn been shown to reduce the need for analgesic drugs with their associated side-effects (Haywood, 1975).

Psychological approaches using hypnosis, relaxation and distraction techniques have also been shown to help reduce procedure-related pain (APM, 2005). Time should also be allowed for patients to consider any information given to them (Heafield, 1999). Practical considerations such as the choice of dressing used on wounds (Ross, 2004) or simply irrigating a wound with warm saline rather than a gauze swab (Hollingsworth, 1997) can be important.

There is no evidence supporting the view that pain diminishes with age (Harkins, 2000); the incidence of painful conditions actually increases rather than decreases with advancing age. Older patients may, however, complain less about pain due to deterioration in sensory function, concerns over addiction to drugs, acceptance of pain being inevitable with ageing, fear over diagnostic tests, cultural unacceptability of showing pain or adverse

---

Box 9.2 Pain assessment tool

0 = No pain
1 = Mild pain
2 = Moderate pain
3 = Severe pain

---

effects of analgesic drugs. Older people also demonstrate age-related changes in medication sensitivity, toxicity and sensitivity (Fine, 2001).

The adoption of a 'start low, go slow' approach to drug prescription and administration is therefore useful with elderly patients. This does not mean that analgesia should be limited; staff in hospital wards and accident and emergency departments have been shown to under-treat older patients with pain (Jones *et al.*, 1996 and Closs *et al.*, 1993).

Uncontrolled or unexpected pain requires reassessment of the diagnosis and consideration of alternative analgesia. Increasing agitation may be a result of poor pain relief, but also of withdrawal of drugs such as alcohol, benzodiazepines and nicotine or deterioration in organ function. It is a misconception that the provision of analgesia to a patient with acute abdominal pain will mask the signs and symptoms of abdominal pathology and should therefore be withheld until a diagnosis has been established (Thomas *et al.*, 2003).

METHODS OF PAIN RELIEF

The critically ill patient may have rapidly changing physiology, which can impact on the effectiveness of analgesia. The incidence of adverse effects in these patients can therefore be difficult to predict. The adoption of an 'initial little and often' approach using short-acting drugs is therefore advisable. This prevents accumulation within the body of drugs or drug metabolites and allows rapid titration of analgesia according to the patient's level of pain. The use of 'as required' or 'PRN' prescription should be avoided, prescription of drugs being subject to regular reassessment of the patient's pain, prompting changes to the analgesic regime as required.

Oral

Administration should be via the simplest route. In many cases this will mean oral administration, but if this is not possible other options are available. Oral analgesics can be given via nasogastric and gastrostomy tubes. A check needs to be made if the formulation being used is suitable for this method, as it may not be possible to crush tablets.

Intramuscular

Repeated intramuscular (i.m.) injections are simple to administer and cheap, but can be painful. They are therefore best avoided. Indwelling intramuscular catheters are available which avoid the pain of repeated needle insertion into the muscle. Intermittent subcutaneous injections may be less painful, but, like i.m. injections, are unsuitable for the needle-phobic patient. Injections are also subject to wide variations in plasma concentration of the drug (Austin *et al.*, 1980), a problem which may be enhanced in patients with shock and reduced peripheral blood supply delaying absorption of the drug from the injected area.

Intravenous

Intravenous (i.v.) injection is both effective and simple to administer. If repeated i.v. injection of strong opioids is required, it may be possible to allow the patient to self-medicate using a patient-controlled analgesia (PCA) pump (Figure 9.2). The advantage of this approach is its good level of patient satisfaction (Chumbley *et al.*, 1998) and reduction in the need for repeated checking of controlled drugs. However, patients should be carefully assessed for their ability to use PCA correctly, as they may be unable to operate the system due to physical disability or cognitive impairment resulting from organ dysfunction or drugs. Continuous infusions of opioids are associated with higher risks of adverse side-effects than PCA (Dawson *et al.*, 1995). They are therefore best avoided unless the patient has a terminal condition or is closely monitored in a critical care area.

Regional analgesia

Sophisticated techniques, such as epidurals and continuous nerve blocks, should be administered by suitably trained personnel

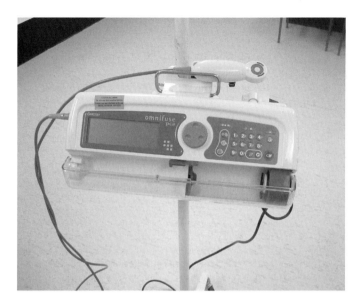

Fig 9.2 Patient Controlled Analgesia (PCA) pump

and their subsequent care provided by staff familiar with the specific needs of the patient. Specialist teams who deal with pain issues should be available in all hospitals in order to provide advice and specialist techniques as and when required (RCA and Pain Society, 2003).

ANALGESICS

Opiates
All opiates broadly have the same effects: an agonist action upon opioid receptors within the body producing the pharmacological effect of analgesia. Therefore, there is little value in giving more than one opiate at a time. If the initial drug dose does not work, the dose and frequency of administration should be checked

before changing to an alternative drug. Initial pain management should be achieved by the regular administration of short-acting drugs taking into consideration any potential adverse effects of the drug being considered.

Morphine is the most commonly used strong opiate for severe pain. Interpatient response can vary greatly, necessitating titration of dose against patient response (Macintyre and Jarvis, 1996). Both morphine and codeine are poorly absorbed orally, which is why oral morphine solution in strengths < 13 mg per 5 ml and oral codeine are not considered controlled drugs. Parenteral administration avoids this problem, but does require a reduction in the dose, being two to three times more potent than an equivalent oral dose.

As well as reducing pain, opiates can induce sedation, nausea and vomiting, itching, constipation euphoria/confusion, retention of urine and respiratory depression. These effects can be reversed by the short-acting opioid antagonist naloxone. Repeat administration may be required if long-acting opiates have been used. The exception to this is buphrenorphine, which is a partial opioid agonist and poorly effected by naloxone. If deep sedation and respiratory depression occur, tracheal intubation and ventilation may be required in order to protect the airway and maintain oxygenation.

The use of strong opioids is often necessary to assist the tolerance of a patient to oral intubation and invasive respiratory support. However, this can also contribute to gastric stasis and constipation with prolonged use.

Morphine has an active metabolite. This can have the same effects as morphine and can accumulate in patients with renal impairment. Fentanyl and oxycodone have the advantage over morphine in that they have relatively inactive metabolites (Mercadante & Arcuri, 2004), making them potentially more suitable for patients with impaired kidney function.

Pethidine (Meperidine) has the potential to induce seizures due to accumulation of its metabolite nor-pethidine. Its use is currently being discouraged in favour of other opioids (Latta *et al.*,

2002) and is not thought to be superior to morphine for the treatment of biliary colic (O'Connor *et al.*, 2000). Tramadol is a weak mu receptor agonist as well as serotonin, and noradrenalin inhibitor. This makes it a useful drug for moderate to severe pain with a low risk of respiratory depression and potential for addiction. It can therefore be of value for use with patients with morbid obesity with obstructive sleep apnoea (Simmonds, 1999). Its inhibitory effects on neurotransmitters also make it potentially useful for neuropathic pain (Duhmke *et al.*, 2004), but can lead to neurotoxic effects in high doses (Sachs, 2005).

Methadone is a potent analgesic, which is commonly used as a heroin substitute for substance abusers. It has a long duration of action and may be used for patients, such as those with cancer, whose pain is difficult to control with more conventional opioids (Twycross *et al.*, 1998). Patients taking methadone should continue to do so when admitted to hospital, or an equipotent substitute given if they are unable to continue taking this orally. When changing from one drug to another, consideration of the relative potencies of each drug should be made in order to prevent under- or overmedication of the patient (see Box 9.3.)

Box 9.3 Conversion values from oral morphine to alternative opiate

- Oxycodone oral — divide by 2
- Tramadaol oral/injection — divide by 4
- Fentanyl — divide by 100 or 150 to give micrograms
- Diamorphine sub cut — divide by 3

These are approximate values only and may differ according to local policy.

Analgesic patches (Fentanyl and Buphrenorphine) have little value in the initial management of acute pain conditions because of slow onset of action. Patients may, however, be admitted to hospital already using them for a chronic pain condition. Advice should be sought regarding their continued use and possible substitution with another drug.

Policies should be in place for the management of opiate-induced nausea and vomiting. In addition, some form of laxative and/or stool softener is frequently required due to the incidence of constipation regardless of the route of administration. All patients receiving strong opiates should undergo regular monitoring for signs of sedation, and respiratory depression.

Paracetamol

Paracetamol is cheap, effective and well tolerated, particularly if given regularly, with the added benefit of antipyretic qualities. It can be given orally, rectally (although absorption is variable) and intravenously.

Direct comparisons between paracetamol and non-steroidal anti-inflammatory drugs (NSAIDs) have shown it to be as effective as NSAIDs in situations such as orthopaedic surgery and tension headache (Sach, 2005). Caution should be exercised in patients with liver impairment.

Non-steroidal anti-inflammatory drugs

NSAIDs are a group of drugs with anti-inflammatory, antipyretic and analgesic effects resulting from the inhibition of the enzyme cyclooxygenase (Cox). This occurs in two forms, types 1 and 2. Cox-1 is important in the production of prostaglandins, which regulate blood clotting, maintenance of gastric mucosa, renal and platelet function. Cox-2 has a more specific role in the inflammatory process.

Older NSAIDs (aspirin and diclofenac) are non-selective, leading to potential side-effects such as gastric irritation, reduction in platelet function and renal function. Only 10–15% of asthmatics are sensitive to NSAIDs. They are therefore not contraindicated in asthmatic patients, but caution should be exercised when prescribing them (West & Fernadez, 2003).

Gastroprotective drugs such as histamine blockers and proton pump blockers may be used to reduce the risk of gastrointestinal haemorrhage when using non-selective NSAIDs.

Cox-2-specific NSAIDs selectively inhibit Cox-2, resulting in fewer side-effects than other NSAIDs. Potential benefits may be offset by an increased risk of thromboembolic events in at-risk patients (FDA, 2004 and www.jr.ox.ac.uk). No NSAIDs, regardless of type, should be given to patients with shock, impaired renal function or dehydration. Clinically, there is little difference in efficacy between individual preparations (Gotze, 2003).

Adjuvants

Adjuvants are a mixed collection of drugs, which do not have a direct analgesic action but may be used to influence the causes of pain. For example, diazepam and baclofen can help reduce painful muscle spasm, with anticonvulsants being used for neuropathic pain. Peritumour oedema can cause pressure and pain in the surrounding tissues: a corticosteroid, e.g. dexamethasone, may be used to help reduce this.

The World Health Organization's 'analgesic ladder' (1986) (originally developed for the management of cancer pain) is a useful approach to the use of all of the above drugs. However, in acute conditions it is often necessary to work down the ladder rather than work up and has been modified by the World Federation of Societies of Anaesthesiologists to include the use of local anaesthetics for severe pain (www.nda.ox.ac.uk Jan 2006).

Local anaesthetics

Local anaesthetics work by blocking sodium channels in nerve cell wall membranes, resulting in inhibition of nerve transmission. Short- and long-acting agents are available, the choice being dependant upon the duration of analgesia required. They may be applied topically as a cream or as a gel prior to i.v. cannula insertion or urinary catheter insertion. Infiltration around a wound site can be done by injection or via a catheter, allowing continuous infusion and prolonged pain relief.

Local anaesthetics are also used to provide epidural and regional nerve blockade. This can be given as a single injection, or via a continuous infusion catheter extending the duration of analgesia. These techniques are most commonly used for post-operative analgesia, the great advantage being the avoidance of strong opiates and their associated effects. Inadvertent i.v. injection can, however, induce toxic effects (Serpall, 2003).

Epidural analgesia is contraindicated in the presence of coagulopathy or recent administration of anticoagulant injections due to the risk of epidural haematoma formation. Small doses of opiates, e.g. diamorphine, morphine or fentanyl, can be added to epidural infusions.

Entonox

Entonox consists of a 50/50 mix of nitrous oxide and oxygen gases and, when inhaled, provides moderate pain relief. Its rapid onset of action and short duration make it particularly useful for procedural pain such as dressing changes, and to augment other types of pain relief. Ideally it should not be used for more than 20 min or in a confined area unless some form of scavenging device is used to remove waste gases.

The gas mixture is also administered via a demand valve under positive pressure, so is contraindicated in patients with pneumothorax, severe bullous emphysema, intestinal obstruction and maxillo-facial fractures (BOC Medical, 2006).

NON-PHARMACEUTICAL METHODS TO PROVIDE PAIN RELIEF

Non-pharmaceutical methods to provide pain relief include:

- Splinting a fracture
- Immobilization if an inflamed joint
- Cooling an area that is inflamed
- Application of therapeutic heat
- Patient reassurance
- Psychological support

- Relaxation therapy
- Transcutaneous electrical nerve stimulation (TENS)
- Aromatherapy
- Acupuncture (Lin *et al.*, 2002).

(Source: Smith, 2003)

The use of TENS may be contraindicated in patients with a pace maker. Acupuncture is contraindicated in patients with bleeding disorders or clotting abnormalities.

PROBLEMS ASSOCIATED WITH PAIN AND ANALGESIC DRUGS

Nausea and vomiting

Nausea and vomiting often accompany pain and occur in 20–30% of patients following surgery (Cohen *et al.*. 1994). They can also result from a variety of other causes, such as the use of analgesic, anaesthetic and chemotherapy drugs, gastric irritation due to food poisoning, gastric distension and bowel obstruction, unpleasant sights and smells, vestibula disturbance causing motion sickness, raised intracranial pressure and hypotension.

When prescribing an anti-emetic, the cause of the problem must first be identified in order that the right type of anti-emetic is prescribed. An alternative intervention, such as the passage of a nasogastric tube or correction of hypotension, may also be required. It should be standard practice to prescribe a suitable anti-emetic when prescribing strong opiates.

Tolerance, dependence and addiction

In the vast majority of patients with genuine acute pain and given adequate levels of pain relief, problems related to addiction are extremely rare. However, patients receiving opiates for long periods can develop tolerance and physical dependence. These, in turn, can pose significant problems for pain management, not just for the patient with a substance abuse problem but also for those taking strong opiates for chronic conditions, who subsequently become critically ill.

Tolerance can occur over time as the body develops a resistance to the effects of the drug. Increasing doses may then be required in order to achieve the desired effect. Dependence manifests as withdrawal effects upon abrupt reduction or cessation of a drug. Symptoms of opiate withdrawal include:

- Agitation
- Abdominal cramps
- Muscle aches and pains
- Nausea and vomiting
- Rhinorrhoea and sneezing
- Trembling
- Diarrhoea.

Prevention of withdrawal involves administration of the normal analgesic or a suitable equipotent replacement. Other analgesics, e.g. paracetamol and NSAIDs, can also be used to treat the patient's pain. If additional opiate analgesia is required, this will be in addition to the maintenance opioid dose and titrated against the patient's response. PCA with a background continuous infusion can be particularly useful for patients who are drug abusers (Jage & Bey, 2000).

Addiction is a psychological dependence upon a drug, features of which are craving for a particular drug(s) and development of withdrawal effects upon cessation of the drug(s) being taken. Treatment of addiction is a specialist field requiring commitment from the patient and is not appropriate in the acute setting. However, much can be done to prevent and reduce the effects of withdrawal symptoms caused by tolerance to drugs in the acute situation, in turn improving patient concordance with medical treatment.

CONCLUSION

Good pain management is a key feature in achieving a favourable outcome for the patient, resulting in fewer physiological and psychological adverse effects. It is also rewarding for staff to be able to manage a patient's discomfort, in turn enhancing their recovery period. The subjective nature of pain and variability in patients' clinical conditions mean that the adoption of a multimodal approach utilizing differing techniques is sometimes required in order to meet individual patient needs. Staff need to be aware of these techniques and either be able to implement them themselves or have access to specialist services for help and support.

REFERENCES

APM (2005) *Acute Pain Management: Scientific Evidence.* Australian and New Zealand College of Anaesthetists and Faculty of Pain Medicine, xv.

Arbor, R. (2000) Sedation and pain management in critically ill adults. *Critical Care Nurse* **20**, 39–56.

Austin, K, Stapleton, J, Mather, L. (1980) Multiple intramuscular injections: a major source of variability in analgesic response to meriperidine. *Pain* **8**, 47.

Bennet, M. (2001) The LANSS Pain Scale: the Leeds assessment of neuropathic symptoms and signs. *Pain*; **92**, 147–157.

Bjordal, J, Johnson, M, Ljunggreen, A. (2003) Transcutaneous electrical nerve stimulation (TENS) can reduce post operative analgesic consumption. A meta-analysis with assessment of optimal treatment parameters for post operative pain. *Eur J Pain* **7**, 181–188.

Blyth, F, March, L, Cousins, M. (2003) Chronic pain related disability and use of analgesia and health services in a Sydney community. *Med J Aust* **179**, 84–87.

BOC Medical (2006) *Entonox: Controlled Pain Relief. A Reference Guide.* BOC, London.

Briggs, M, & Closs, J. (1999) A descriptive study of visual analogue scales and verbal rating scales for the assessment of post operative pain in orthopaedic patients. *J Pain Symptom Manage* **18**, 438–446.

BNF (2006) *British National Formulary.*

Chumbley, G, Hall, G, Salmon, P. (1998) Patient controlled analgesia: an assessment by 200 patients. *Anaesthesia* **53**, 216–221.

Closs, S, Fairlough, H, Tierney, A, Currie, E. (2003) Pain in elderly orthopaedic patients. *Journal of Clinical Nursing* **2**, 41–45.

Cohen, M, Duncan, P, De Boer, D. (1994) The preoperative interview: assessing risk factors for nausea and vomiting. *Anaesthesia and Analgesia* **78**, 7–16.

Cousins, M, Brennan, F, Carr, D. (2004) Editorial: Pain relief: a universal human right. *Pain* **112**, 1–4.

Dawson, P, Libreri, F, Jones, D *et al.* (1995) The efficacy of adding a continuous intravenous morphine infusion to patient controlled analgesia (PCA) in abdominal surgery *Anesthesia and Intensive Care* **23**, 453–458.

Dumhke, R, Cornblath, D, Hollingshead, J. (2004) *Tramadol for neuropathic pain.* The Cochrane Data Base of Systematic reviews, Issue 2 Art No: CD =003726.

FDA (2004) *FDA Public Health Advisory: Safety of Vioxx.* US Food and Drug Administration.

Fine, P. (2001) Opioid analgesic drugs in older people. *Clinics in Geriatric Medicine* **17**, 479–487.

Frank, J.D, & Frank J.B. (1991) *Persuasion and Healing*, 3rd edn. John Hopkins University Press, Baltimore, MD.

Gotze, P. (2003) Non steroidal anti-inflammatory drugs. *Clinical Evidence* **9**, 1292–1300.

Harkins, S. (2000) Aging and pain. In: Loeser, J, Chapman, C, Butler, S, eds. *Bonicas Management of Pain,* 3rd edn. Williams and Wilkins, Baltimore, MD.

Jones, J, Johnson, K, McNich, M. (1996) Age as a risk factor for inadequate emergency department analgesia. *Am J Emerg Med* **14**, 151–160.

Haywood, J. (1975) *Information: A Prescription Against Pain.* RCN, London.

Heafield, R.H. (1999) The management of procedural pain. *Professional Nurse* **15**, 127–129.

Hollingsworth, H. (1997) Wound care – less pain, more gain. *Nursing Times* **93**, 89–91.

Jage, J, & Bey, T. (2000) Post operative analgesia in patients with substance use disorders: Part 1. *Acute Pain* **3**, 140–155.

JCAHA + NPC (2001) *Pain: Current Understanding of Assessment, Management and Treatments.* Joint Commission on Accreditation of Health Care Organisations and the National Pharmaceutical Council Inc. Available at http://www.fleshandbones.com/readingroom/viewchapter.cfm?ID=1512/ Last accessed Mar. 2007

Latta, K, Ginsberg, B, Barkin, R *et al.* (2002) Meperidine: a critical review. *Am J Ther* **9**, 53–68.

Lin, J, Lo, M, Wen, Y *et al.* (2002) The effect of high and low frequency electroaccupuncture in pain following lower abdominal surgery. *Pain* **99**, 509–514.

Macintyre, P, & Jarvis, D. (1996) Age is the best predictor of post operative morphine requirements. *Pain* **64**, 357–367.

Mercandante, S, & Arcuri E. (2004) Opioids and renal function. *Journal of Pain* **5**, 2–19.

Merskey, H. (1979) Pain terms: a list with definitions and notes on usage. Recommended by the Subcommittee on Taxonomy. *Pain* **6**, 249–252.

Melzack, R, & Wall, P. (1965) Pain mechanisms: a new theory. *Science* **150**, 971–979.

O'Connor, A, Schug, J, Cardwell, H. (2000) A comparison of the efficacy and safety of morphine and pethidine for suspected renal colic in the emergency setting. *J Accid Emerg Med* **17**, 261–264.

RCA and Pain Society (2003) Pain management services – good practice. Available at www.rcoa.ac.uk Last accessed Mar. 2007.

Ross, S. (2004) Surgical wound care: current views on minimising dressing-related pain. *Professional Nurse* **20**, 38.

Sach, C. (2005) www.aafp.org/afp20050301/913 Last accessed Jan. 2006.

Serpall, M. (2003) Clinical pharmacology – local anaesthetics. In: Rowbotham, DJ, & Macintyre, PE, eds. *Acute Pain*, Chapter 5. Arnold, London.

Simmonds, T. (1999) Surgical treatment of morbid obesity. *Professional Nurse* **15,** 109–121.

Smith, G. (2003) *ALERT Acute Life-Threatening Events Recognition and Treatment,* 2nd edn. University of Portsmouth, Portsmouth.

Thomas, S, Sien, W, Cheema, F *et al.* (2003) Effects of morphine analgesia in diagnostic accuracy in emergency department patients with abdominal pain: a prospective, randomised trial. *J Am Coll Surg* **196,** 18–31.

Turk, D. (1995) Biopsychosocial perspective on chronic pain. In: Gatchel, R, & Turk, D, eds. *Psychological Approaches to Pain Management.* Guildford Press, New York.

Twycross, R, Wilcock, A, Thorp, S. (1998) *Palliative Care Formulary.* Radcliffe, Oxford.

West, P, & Fernadez, C. (2003) Safety of Cox 2 inhibitors in asthma patients with aspirin sensitivity. *Ann Pharmacother* **37,** 1497–1501.

WHO (1986) *Cancer Pain Relief.* WHO, Geneva. www.nda.ox.ac.uk. Last accessed Jan. 2007.

10 | Ethical Issues in Critical Care

INTRODUCTION

The primary aim of medical treatment is to benefit the patient by restoring or maintaining health as far as possible, thereby maximizing benefit and minimizing harm (Jevon, 2001). If treatment fails or ceases to be beneficial, or if an adult, competent patient refuses treatment, the aim of medical treatment cannot be realised and the justification for providing it is removed (BMA *et al.*, 2001). In the critically ill patient, ethical issues can arise which require rapid decisions to be made relating to those issues.

However, the traditional paternalistic approach to the delivery of healthcare, in which the medical and nursing staff 'know best', is no longer suitable, because patients have a right to be consulted; in fact, doctors and nurses are usually no more likely to be morally or ethically correct than other members of society, even though they possess more in-depth knowledge of the medical subject matter (Smith, 2003). The nurse must respect the patient's autonomy, his right to decide whether or not to undergo any healthcare intervention; the nurse has a professional responsibility to ensure that the best interests and well-being of the patient are always promoted and safeguarded (NMC, 2004).

The aim of this chapter is to provide an overview of ethical issues in critical care.

LEARNING OBJECTIVES

At the end of this chapter the reader will be able to:

❏ List the four moral principles of ethics
❏ Discuss the importance of advanced directives

❏ Discuss the procedure for 'do not attempt resuscitation' orders

❏ Outline the procedure when withholding or withdrawing treatment.

FOUR MORAL PRINCIPLES OF ETHICS
The four moral principles of ethics are:

• Respect for autonomy
• Beneficence
• Non-maleficence
• Justice.

(Beauchamp & Childress, 1994 and Smith, 2003)

Respect for autonomy
The principle of respect for autonomy is the right of a fully informed patient to choose a certain course of action for himself (Smith, 2003), rather than being subjected to a paternalistic decision being made by the medical and nursing professions (Baskett *et al.*, 2005).

Autonomy requires that the patient is adequately informed, competent, free from undue pressure and that there is consistency in the preferences of the patient (Baskett *et al.*, 2005). An adequately informed decision requires that the patient receives and understands accurate information concerning his condition and prognosis, the nature of the proposed intervention, together with alternatives, risks and benefits (American Heart Association, 2005).

The principle of autonomy has been endorsed in recent times with the introduction of such legislation as the Human Rights Act (Resuscitation Council UK, 2006). It has also been endorsed by the Nursing and Midwifery Council (NMC, 2004).

Beneficence
The principle of beneficence implies that the healthcare practitioner must provide healthcare to the patient while balancing

potential benefits and risks (Baskett *et al.*, 2005). Although this has been traditionally viewed as preserving life, in some situations where the patient's quality of life is poor, e.g. severe pain or disability, death may be more beneficial for the patient.

Non-maleficence

The principle of non-maleficence means doing no harm (primum non nocere) (Smith, 2003 and Baskett *et al.*, 2005). A conflict can arise if a beneficial medical intervention (e.g. pain relief in terminal illness) has a potential risk of harming the patient (e.g. respiratory depression) (Smith, 2003).

Justice

The principle of justice implies a duty to spread benefits and risks equally within a population (Baskett *et al.*, 2005), i.e. equity (fairness) and equality (equal access for everyone) (Smith, 2003).

IMPORTANCE OF ADVANCED DIRECTIVES

An advanced directive is a method of communicating the patient's wishes concerning his future care, particularly towards the end of his life, and must be expressed while he is mentally competent and not under duress (Baskett *et al.*, 2005). Refusal of treatment does not need to be in writing for it to be valid; if the patient has expressed clear and consistent refusal verbally, this is then likely to have the same status as a written advanced directive (Resuscitation Council UK, 2006).

An advance directive is legally binding as long as the adult patient:

- Intended it to apply in the circumstances
- Was mentally competent at the time it was made
- Was not under the influence of someone else at the time
- Was fully aware of the relevant risks and complications.

(Resuscitation Council UK, 2000)

In complying, the doctor must be satisfied that the advanced directive is genuine and applies to the current situation.

Difficulties can be encountered if the document is not immediately available, if the patient has second thoughts when facing imminent death and in the emergency situation (Resuscitation Council UK, 2006). The patient should clearly stipulate the situation envisaged when life support should be withheld or discontinued (Baskett *et al.*, 2005). In addition, the patient must ensure that both the healthcare team and his relatives are aware of his wishes if they are to be implemented (Resuscitation Council UK, 2006): his medical notes can then be updated appropriately, following local protocols.

DO NOT ATTEMPT RESUSCITATION ORDERS

Although modern resuscitation techniques have resulted in the successful resuscitation of many patients, they unfortunately have also made it possible to bring 'dead' patients back to life, prolong the process of dying and deny patients dignified and peaceful deaths with their loved ones present. 'You can treat and must not kill, but do not try to bring a dead soul back to life' (Pinder, 5th century BC, cited in Negovsky, 1993).

It is therefore 'essential to identify patients for whom cardiopulmonary arrest represents a terminal event in their illness and in whom CPR is inappropriate. It is also essential to identify those patients who do not want CPR to be attempted and who competently refuse it' (BMA *et al.*, 2001).

Decisions Relating to Cardiopulmonary Resuscitation, a joint statement from the British Medical Association, Resuscitation Council (UK) and the Royal College of Nursing (2001), outlines the ethical and legal standards for planning patient care and decision making in relation to cardiopulmonary resuscitation (CPR).

The Human Rights Act 1998 and DNAR orders

The Human Rights Act 1998 incorporates the majority of the rights set out in the European Convention on Human Rights into UK law. In order to meet their obligations under the Act, health professionals must be able to demonstrate that their decisions are compatible with the human rights identified in the Articles of the

Convention (Resuscitation Council UK, 2000). Provisions particularly relevant to Do Not Attempt Resuscitation (DNAR) orders include the right to:

- Life (Article 2)
- Be free from inhuman or degrading treatment (Article 3)
- Respect for privacy and family life (Article 8)
- Freedom of expression (Article 10)
- Be free from discriminatory practices in respect of these rights (Article 14).

(BMA *et al.*, 2001)

Factors to consider when discussing a DNAR order

The following factors should be considered when discussing a DNAR order:

- The likely clinical outcome of CPR, including the chances of successfully restarting the patient's heart and breathing, and the overall benefit achieved from a successful CPR
- The patient's known or ascertainable wishes – these are an essential element in the decision
- The patient's human rights, including the right to life and the right to be free from degrading treatment.

(BMA *et al.*, 2001)

Who should make the order

The consultant or GP in charge of the patient's care is ultimately responsible for making a DNR order (BMA *et al.*, 2001). If the consultant is not available, their deputy can make the decision. However, the consultant must be informed at the earliest opportunity. The views of other members of the healthcare team should also be sought.

Nurses have traditionally left DNAR decisions to medical colleagues; it is perhaps deemed easier to follow medical orders than be the patient's advocate and take on board their values and wishes (Ellis, 1991). However, the nurse must always act in such a manner as to promote and safeguard the interests and well-being of the patient, recognize his autonomy and respect the uniqueness and dignity of each patient (NMC, 2004). Therefore if the nurse considers that CPR is inappropriate for a patient, or is aware that the patient does not wish to be resuscitated in the event of a cardiopulmonary arrest, then she should raise the issue with senior medical staff at the earliest opportunity.

Role of the patient

The patient's rights are central to decision making on resuscitation; he has as much right to be involved in a DNAR order as he does with other decisions about his care and treatment (Department of Health, 2000). Most patients would prefer to discuss the issue of CPR and there are often inconsistencies between what the patient wants and what the medical staff thinks the patient wants (Broekman, 1998). A competent patient should understand that he is entitled to have an opportunity to discuss CPR if he wishes to; in addition, when a DNAR order is based on considerations related to quality of life, his views are particularly important (BMA *et al.*, 2001).

There are clearly situations where sensitive exploration of the patient's wishes should be undertaken, e.g. a patient in the latter stages of a terminal illness who is at risk of having a cardiopulmonary arrest. However, some patients may object to a DNAR order and request that CPR is carried out even though it is not in their best interests and will not benefit them. It is important to secure an understanding and acceptance of the clinical judgement. However, if the patient still requests that a DNAR order is not made, then this should be respected (BMA *et al.*, 2001). 'Doctors cannot be required to give treatment contrary to their clinical judgement, but should, whenever possible, respect the patient's wishes to receive treatment which carries only a very small chance of success or benefit' (BMA *et al.*, 2001).

Sometimes it will not be possible to consult the patient, e.g. if the patient is unconscious. In England, Wales and Northern Ireland no person can legally give consent to medical treatment on behalf of an adult who is incapacitated. Medical staff have the authority to act in the best interests of the patient when consent is not available (BMA *et al.*, 2001). In Scotland the Adults with Incapacity Act permits people over the age of 16 to appoint a proxy decision maker, who then has the legal power to grant consent to medical treatment if the patient becomes incapacitated, as long as it is not judged to be against the best interests of the patient (Jevon, 2001).

Role of the patient's close relatives

It is good practice to involve the patient's close relatives, although their views have no legal status in the decision-making process; a competent patient's consent should first be obtained and any refusal to allow information to be disclosed to family or friend should be respected (Jevon, 2001). In addition, wherever possible, patients should be asked in advance who they want, or do not want, to be involved in DNAR order making if they become incapacitated (BMA *et al.*, 2001).

If the patient is unable to express a view, e.g. due to unconsciousness, the opinion of his close relatives may be sought regarding his best interests. People close to the patient may be able to comment on the patient's wishes and quality of life. However, it must be clarified that their role is to reflect the views of the patient, not to take decisions on behalf of the patient (BMA *et al.*, 2001).

Documentation of a DNAR order

When a DNAR order is made, it must be clearly documented in the patient's notes by the most senior clinician present, following locally agreed guidelines. To avoid all confusion the phrase 'not for attempted cardiopulmonary resuscitation' should be used (BMA *et al.*, 2001). The entry should be signed, dated and should include the rationale behind the order, who was consulted and when it should be reviewed. If the patient's circumstances (e.g. prognosis, expressed wishes) change and the DNR decision is perhaps no longer appropriate, nursing staff should bring this to the attention of medical colleagues as soon as possible and ensure that it is reviewed.

A DNAR order must also be documented in the nursing notes by the primary nurse or most senior member of the nursing team whose responsibility it is to communicate the decision to other members of the nursing team. It would be advisable for the nurse to check that what has actually been written in the medical notes clearly reflects the conversation concerning the DNAR order, as misunderstandings can occur. Accurate record keeping is essential; it will help to protect the welfare of the patient by promoting better communication and dissemination of information between members of the inter-professional healthcare team (NMC, 2005).

Communication of a DNAR order

Effective communication will help to avoid misunderstanding and unnecessary anxiety. When a DNAR order has been made on clinical grounds, discussion with the patient and relatives should be aimed at securing an understanding and acceptance of the clinical decision. A DNAR order only applies to CPR. It should be made clear that all other treatment and care which are appropriate for the patient are not precluded and will not be influenced by a DNAR decision. The DNAR policy should be readily available to those who may wish to consult it, including patients, relatives and carers (Department of Health, 2000).

Sometimes it is not possible for relatives to be consulted when a DNAR decision is made, e.g. if they are on holiday and not contactable. However, nursing staff should ensure that relatives are informed at the earliest opportunity.

When a DNAR order has been made, it must be effectively communicated to all relevant healthcare professionals, including medical staff, nursing staff, locum and agency staff.

DNAR policy

The Joint Statement (BMA *et al.*, 2001) stresses that their 'guidelines should be viewed as a framework providing basic principles within which decisions regarding local policies on CPR may be formulated'. Individual Trusts and hospitals should produce their own DNAR policy based on these guidelines, but take into account local circumstances, e.g. the GP may be responsible for the patient. The use of a flow chart (Figure 10.1) is helpful for staff to follow when considering a DNAR order.

PROCEDURE FOR WITHHOLDING OR WITHDRAWING TREATMENT

If treatment fails or ceases to be beneficial, or if an adult, competent patient refuses treatment, the aim of medical treatment cannot be realized and the justification for providing it is removed (BMA *et al.*, 2001). Withholding or withdrawing treatment will then need to be considered. This is usually when brainstem death has been confirmed or when the patient's quality of life is judged to be poor and there is no prospect of a return to a quality of life acceptable to the patient (Smith, 2003).

If brainstem death has been confirmed (Box 10.1), withholding or withdrawing treatment is relatively straightforward. However, if the brainstem is intact but the function of the cerebral cortex has ceased due to ischaemic damage, e.g. following a prolonged cardiopulmonary resuscitation or due to a cerebral injury, such as head injury, the patient's life can be prolonged because spontaneous ventilation is still possible even in the absence of cognitive function; this situation is called a persistent vegetative state, and withdrawing treatment in these patients is very difficult because prognosis is uncertain (Leach, 2004).

When considering the decision to withhold or withdraw treatment, the following factors should be taken into account:

- The patient's wishes
- Diagnosis
- Severity of disease and co-existing illnesses
- Prognosis
- Response to current treatment

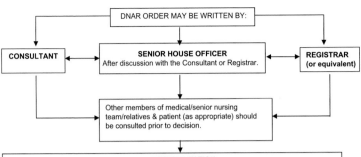

DNAR ORDER MAY BE WRITTEN BY:

CONSULTANT

SENIOR HOUSE OFFICER
After discussion with the Consultant or Registrar.

REGISTRAR
(or equivalent)

Other members of medical/senior nursing team/relatives & patient (as appropriate) should be consulted prior to decision.

DOCUMENTATION

- 'Not For Attempted Cardiopulmonary Resuscitation' should be documented legibly in the medical & nursing notes along with the date & time of the order being made.
- If written by the SHO, the name of the Consultant or Registrar who has agreed the DNAR order should be documented in the medical notes.
- The name of the clinician writing the order should be printed clearly and signed.
- Reason for the order and any discussions undertaken with the patient or relatives should be documented. If it is inappropriate to discuss the decision with either the patient and/or relatives, the reason for this should be clearly documented.
- If specific review times are inappropriate the reasons for this should be documented along with the next review time. Also, the name of the Consultant or Registrar who has agreed to different review times should be recorded if written by the SHO.
- Complete blue Resuscitation Checklist form and place at the front of the medical notes.

COMMUNICATION

Ensure that the decision is communicated to:
- other relevant health professionals
- relatives and patients as appropriate.

REVIEW

The DNAR order should be reviewed and re-recorded (in medical notes and on blue Resuscitation Checklist form):
- **within 72 hours** at the Manor
- **on transfer** to the care of another Consultant, or Hospital
- **at the discretion of the Consultant or Registrar involved with the order (refer to Documentation box)**

DNAR ORDER APPLIES UNTIL IT IS REVIEWED & RE-CONFIRMED, AND FOR THE DURATION OF THAT HOSPITAL ADMISSION ONLY

Fig 10.1 Flow chart for making a DNAR order (Walsall Hospitals NHS Trust)

Box 10.1 Brain stem function tests

- Performed > 6–24 h following the precipitating event
- Undertaken by two doctors who are not part of the transplant team, one a consultant; both should be registered > 5 years; two sets of function tests should be performed, either separately or together.
- Six legally required findings to establish brainstem function death: absent papillary, corneal, vestibule-ocular and gag/cough reflexes, no cranial nerve motor responses in response to painful stimuli and apnoea when the ventilator is disconnected despite a $PaCO_2$ > 6.7 kPa.

(Source: Leach, 2004)

- Physiological reserve
- Anticipated quality of life for the patient.

(Smith, 2003)

If treatment is withheld or withdrawn, protocols should be in place to ensure that the patient's comfort and dignity are maintained (Leach, 2004).

CONCLUSION

There are a number of ethical issues that can arise when caring for an acutely ill patient. It is important to ensure that the patient's rights are central to any decisions that are made, particularly in relation to DNAR orders. The nurse has a professional responsibility to adhere to professional standards stipulated by the NMC (2004).

REFERENCES

American Heart Association (2005) 2005 American Heart Association guidelines for cardiopulmonary resuscitation and emergency cardiovascular care: Part IV-6 Part 2: Ethical issues. *Circulation* **112,** Supplement.

Basket, P, Steen, P, Bossaert, L. (2005) European Resuscitation Council Guidelines for Resuscitation 2005 Section 8: The ethics of resuscitation and end-of-life decisions. *Resuscitation* **67S1,** S171–180.

Beauchamp, T, & Childress, J, eds. (1994) *Principles of Biomedical Ethics,* 3rd edn. Oxford University Press, Oxford.

British Medical Association, Resuscitation Council UK, Royal College of Nursing (2001) *Decisions Relating to Cardiopulmonary Resuscitation. A Joint Statement from the British Medical Association, The Resuscitation Council UK and The Royal College Of Nursing.* BMA, London.

British Medical Association (2000) *The Impact of the Human Rights Act 1998 on Medical Decision Making.* BMA, London.

Broekman, B. (1998) Discussing resuscitation with patients, why not? *Resuscitation* **37,** 2062.

Department of Health (2000) Health Service Circular: *Resuscitation Policy.* Department of Health, London.

Jevon, P. (2001) A matter of life and death. *Nursing Times* **97,** 32–33.

NMC (2004) *The NMC Code of Professional Conduct: Standards for Conduct, Performance and Ethics.* NMC, London.

NMC (2005) *Guidelines for Records and Record Keeping.* NMC, London.

Pindar (5th Century BC) cited from Negovsky, VA (1993) Death, dying and revival: ethical aspects. *Resuscitation* **25,** 99–107.

Resuscitation Council (UK) (2006) *Advanced Life Support,* 5th edn. Resuscitation Council UK, London.

APPENDIX

For further information about developments following the publication of the Joint Statement, contact:

Medical Ethics Department, British Medical Association, BMA House, Tavistock Square, London WC1H 9JP; tel 020 7383 6286

Resuscitation Council (UK), 5th Floor, Tavistock House North, Tavistock Square, London WC1H 9HR; tel 020 7388 4678

Royal College of Nursing, 20 Cavendish Square, London W1 OAB; tel 020 7409 3333.

11 | Principles of Good Record Keeping

INTRODUCTION

Good record keeping is a fundamental part of nursing (NMC, 2005). An accurate written record detailing all aspects of nursing the critical ill patient is important, not only because it forms an integral part of the nursing management of the patient, but also because it can help to protect the nurse if defence of her actions is required. The Clinical Negligence Scheme for Trusts (CNST) also requires its members to maintain high standards of record keeping (Dimond, 2005).

The aim of this chapter is to help understand the principles of good record keeping, with specific reference to *Guidelines for Records and Record Keeping* (NMC, 2005).

LEARNING OBJECTIVES

At the end of the chapter the reader will be able to:

❏ Discuss the importance of good record keeping
❏ List the common deficiencies of record keeping
❏ Outline the principles of good record keeping
❏ Outline the importance of auditing patients' records
❏ Discuss the legal issues associated with record keeping.

IMPORTANCE OF GOOD RECORD KEEPING

'Record keeping is an integral part of nursing, midwifery and health visiting practice. It is a tool of professional practice and one that should help the care process. It is not separate from this process and it is not an optional extra to be fitted in if circumstances allow' (NMC, 2005).

Good record keeping will help to protect the welfare of both the patient and practitioner by promoting:

- High standards of clinical care
- Continuity of care
- Better communication and dissemination of information between members of the inter-professional healthcare team (Figure 11.1)
- The ability to detect problems, such as changes in the patient's condition at an early stage

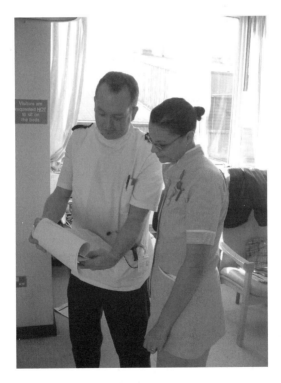

Fig 11.1 Good record keeping will help ensure better communication and dissemination of information between members of the inter-professional healthcare team

- An accurate account of treatment and care planning and delivery.

The quality of record keeping is also a reflection of the standard of nursing practice: good record keeping is an indication that the practitioner is professional and skilled, whereas poor record keeping often highlights wider problems with the individual's practice (NMC, 2005).

COMMON DEFICIENCIES IN RECORD KEEPING

Nearly every report published by the Health Service Commissioner (Health Service Ombudsman) following a complaint identifies examples of poor record keeping that has either hampered the care the patient has received or has made it difficult for healthcare professionals to defend their practice (Dimond, 2005).

Common deficiencies in record keeping encountered include:

- Absence of clarity
- Failure to record action taken when a problem has been identified
- Missing information
- Spelling mistakes
- Inaccurate records.

(Dimond, 2005)

PRINCIPLES OF GOOD RECORD KEEPING

There are a number of factors that underpin good record keeping. The patient's records should:

- Be factual, consistent and accurate
- Be updated as soon as possible after any recordable event
- Provide current information on the care and condition of the patient
- Be documented clearly and in such a way that the text can not be erased
- Be consecutive and accurately dated, timed and signed (including a printed signature)

- Have any alterations and additions dated, timed and signed; all original entries should be clearly legible
- Not include abbreviations, jargon, meaningless phrases, irrelevant speculation and offensive subjective statements
- Still be legible if photocopied
- Identify any problems identified and, most importantly, the action taken to rectify them.

It is important to record all aspects of patient care. Dates and times should be clearly visible and standard coloured ink following local protocols should be used. In particular, it is important to include interventions and any response to the interventions.

Best practice – record keeping

Records must be:
factual
legible
clear
concise
accurate
signed
timed
dated
(Drew *et al.*, 2000)

IMPORTANCE OF AUDITING PATIENTS' RECORDS

Audit can play an important role in ensuring quality of healthcare. In particular, it can help to improve the process of record keeping. By auditing patients' records, the standard can be evaluated and any areas for improvement and staff development identified. Audit tools should be developed at a local level to monitor the standards of record keeping.

Audit should primarily be aimed at serving the interests of the patient rather than the organization (NMC, 2005). A system of peer review may also be of value. Whatever audit system is used, the confidentiality of patients' information applies to audit just as it does to record keeping.

LEGAL ISSUES ASSOCIATED WITH RECORD KEEPING

The patient's records are occasionally required as evidence before a court of law, by the Health Service Commissioner or in order to investigate a complaint at a local level. Sometimes they may be requested by the Nursing and Midwifery Council's Fitness to Practice committees when investigating complaints related to misconduct. Care plans, diaries and anything that makes reference to the patient's care may be required as evidence (NMC, 2005).

What constitutes a legal document is often a cause for concern. Any document requested by the court becomes a legal document (Dimond, 1994), e.g. nursing records, medical records, X-rays, laboratory reports, observation charts – in fact any document which may be relevant to the case.

If any of the documents are missing, the writer of the records may be cross-examined as to the circumstances of their disappearance (Dimond, 1994). 'Medical records are not proof of the truth of the facts stated in them but the maker of the records may be called to give evidence as to the truth as to what is contained in them' (Dimond, 1994).

The approach to record keeping which courts of law adopt tends to be that if it is not recorded, it has not been undertaken (NMC, 2005). Professional judgement is required when deciding what is relevant and what needs to be recorded, particularly if the patient's clinical condition is apparently unchanging and no record has been made of the care that has been delivered.

A registered nurse has both a professional and a legal duty of care. Consequently, when keeping records it is important to be able to demonstrate that:

- A comprehensive nursing assessment of the patient has been undertaken including care that has been planned and provided

- Relevant information is included together with any measures that have been taken in response to changes in the patient's condition
- The duty of care owed to the patient has been honoured and no acts or omissions have compromised the patient's safety
- Arrangements have been made for ongoing care of the patient.

The registered nurse is also accountable for any delegation of record keeping to members of the multi-professional team who are not registered practitioners. For example, if record keeping is delegated to a pre-registration student nurse or a healthcare assistant, competence to perform the task must be ensured and adequate supervision provided. All such entries must be countersigned.

The Access to Health Records Act 1990 gives patients the right of access to their manually maintained health records which were made after 1 November 1991. The Data Protection Act 1998 gives patients the right to access their computer-held records. The Freedom of Information Act 2000 grants the rights to anyone to all information that is not covered by the Data Protection Act 1998 (NMC, 2005).

Sometimes it is necessary to withhold information if it could affect the physical or mental well-being of the patient or if it would breach another patient's confidentiality (NMC, 2005). If the decision to withhold information is made, justification for doing so must be clearly recorded in the patient's notes.

CONCLUSION

When monitoring a critically ill patient it is important to ensure good record keeping. Good record keeping is both the product of good teamwork and an important tool in promoting high-quality healthcare.

REFERENCES

Dimond, B. (1994) *Legal Aspects in Midwifery*. Books for Midwives. Midwifery Press, Cheshire.

Dimond, B. (2005) Exploring common deficiencies that occur in record keeping. *British Journal of Nursing* **14,** 568–570.

Drew, D, Jevon, P, Raby, M. (2000) *Resuscitation of the Newborn.* Butterworth Heinemann, Oxford.

NMC (2005) Guidelines for Records and Record Keeping. NMC, London.

Index